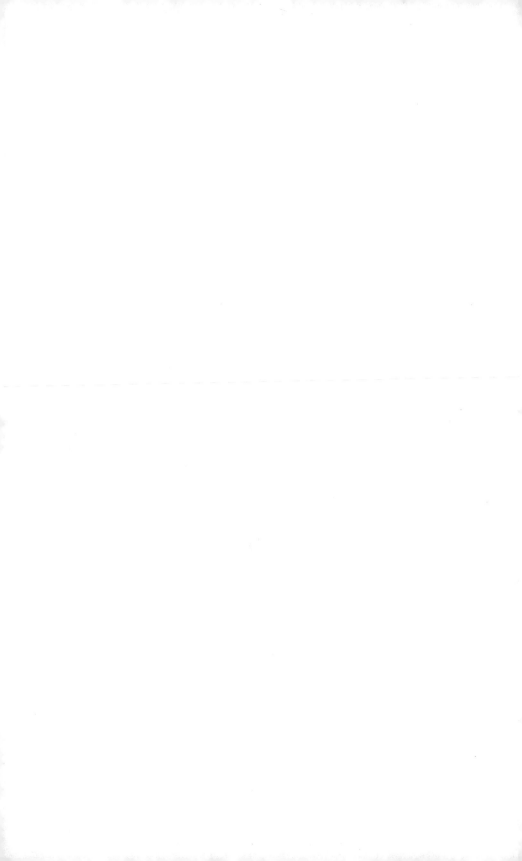

GETTING PHYSICAL

Culture America

Erika Doss
Philip J. Deloria
Series Editors

Karal Ann Marling
Editor Emerita

GETTING
PHYSICAL

THE RISE OF
FITNESS CULTURE
IN AMERICA

SHELLY McKENZIE

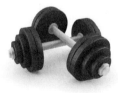

 UNIVERSITY PRESS OF KANSAS

Published by the University
Press of Kansas (Lawrence,
Kansas 66045), which was
organized by the Kansas
Board of Regents and is
operated and funded by
Emporia State University,
Fort Hays State University,
Kansas State University,
Pittsburg State University,
the University of Kansas,
and Wichita State
University

Library of Congress Cataloging-in-Publication Data
McKenzie, Shelly.
Getting physical : the rise of fitness culture in America /
Shelly McKenzie.
    pages cm. — (CultureAmerica)
Includes bibliographical references and index.
ISBN 978-0-7006-1906-1 (cloth : alk. paper)
    1. Physical fitness—United States—History. 2. Exercise—
United States—History. I. Title.
GV510.U5M45   2013
613.7—dc23
                                                    2012049235

British Library Cataloguing-in-Publication Data is
available.

Printed in the United States of America
10 9 8 7 6 5 4 3 2 1

The paper used in this publication is recycled and contains
30 percent postconsumer waste. It is acid free and meets
the minimum requirements of the American National
Standard for Permanence of Paper for Printed Library
Materials Z39.48–1992.

CONTENTS

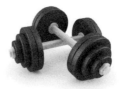

ACKNOWLEDGMENTS

This project has benefited from the expertise and kindness of many individuals. At the University Press of Kansas I've been fortunate to work with a wonderful team. Nancy Scott Jackson took an interest in this project in its earliest form, Ranjit Arab shepherded the initial manuscript to book form, and Fred Woodward saw it through to the end. I'd also like to thank Philip Deloria for his kind words and insightful comments as well as the press's anonymous reviewers who commented on the manuscript.

I owe a huge debt, and at least a ream of paper, to Ellen L. Berg, who read every page in this book, sometimes more than once, and whose friendship, comments, and questions helped see it to completion. My writing courses on food and the body provided an intellectual space to test-drive many of the ideas in this book. Thanks to my supportive colleagues in the Writing Program at George Washington University and the curious and motivated students who thought through what it means to be fit in contemporary America with me in class.

Without the encouragement of Melani McAlister, Chad Heap, and Barney Mergen, my ideas would still be just that. Melani taught me that cultural criticism is a useful tool in the pursuit of social justice. From the start she believed that the history of exercise was a topic worth exploring and that I would be able to do it justice. Chad's attention to detail taught me to be a better historian and a better writer. Barney has been a presence in my intellectual life since my first day of graduate school. Although he has left the concrete jungle of Washington for greener pastures, our friendship endures. I am especially grateful for the support he provided during the book's final stages.

The challenges of doing research in recent history, especially in a field that often leaves a scant paper trail, forced me, in many cases, to pursue documents in places that receive few visits from historians. I am therefore especially grateful to those people and organizations that so generously granted me access to their workplaces and document collections. My thanks to the American Running Association (formerly the National Jogging Association), particularly Barbara Baldwin, and the Road Runners

Club of America, especially Ed Demoney, former acting director. Both organizations allowed me access to their staff libraries, photocopiers, and files, which provided invaluable information related to the early history of the jogging movement. I am also grateful to Primedia Business Magazines and Media, publisher of *Fitness Business Pro*, which publicized my project on its website and helped put me in touch with several longtime members of the fitness industry, resulting in useful oral history interviews and documents. John Firth was one of those who responded, sharing with me a veritable treasure trove of materials on his mother, midcentury television exercise personality Margaret Firth.

Katie Dishman and Kendra Malinowski, of General Mills Archives, provided me with a much-desired Wheaties Sports Fitness Tester and the permission to reprint it. Lara Friedman-Shedlov of the Kautz Family YMCA Archives at the University of Minnesota made my visit there a productive one, and Ryan Bean provided help when it came time for photographs. Carol Bohannon was eager to discuss her father and jogging with me and graciously provided photographs. For additional research assistance, my thanks to Ann Trevor, Scott Daniels of the Oregon Historical Society, Michelle Romero of Northeastern University Archives, and the Air Force History Office. The College of Physicians of Philadelphia and the Cosmos Club Foundation both provided financial support for this project. Sections of chapters 2 and 3 previously appeared in an abridged form in *Women, Wellness, and the Media* (Cambridge Scholars Press, 2008) and are published here with the permission of Cambridge Scholars Publishing.

I owe a tremendous debt to my husband Jim, who has lived with this project since the idea first came to me in a middle-of-the-night lightbulb moment. As a non-gym exerciser, he has endured more fitness talk than he'd care to. He supported this project in all its forms, in every way possible. "Thanks" doesn't even begin to cover it.

GETTING PHYSICAL

INTRODUCTION

FITNESS IN AMERICAN CULTURE

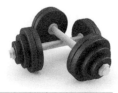

In 1957, physician Donald Dukelow, a member of the American Medical Association's Bureau of Health Education and an adviser to the President's Council on Youth Fitness, noted that although research on exercise was being conducted, "these investigators rarely say whether the observed phenomena are beneficial, harmful, or of no consequence."[1] Just twenty-some years later, expert opinion on exercise had changed drastically. In 1978, the American College of Sports Medicine declared that regular exercise three to five times per week was necessary for the maintenance of good health.[2] By 1988, 10.5 million Americans belonged to health clubs, and the sale of apparel and footwear; exercise books, tapes, and equipment; and gym memberships constituted a multibillion-dollar business.[3] Today, messages about the value of exercise—for both health and appearance—are ubiquitous. From Michelle Obama's "Let's Move" campaign and government warnings about the financial implications of obesity to *The Biggest Loser* and fitness magazines, physical activity is promoted as the answer to the obesity problem, the path to a perfect body, and the ultimate fountain of youth. But how did we get here? Where did modern exercise culture come from? What forces taught us that fitness is an appropriate use of leisure time? What prompted us to take up jogging? To join a gym? To Zumba?

This book explores the foundations of the modern fitness movement. Beginning in the 1950s, Americans were faced with a problem: how could they enjoy the fruits of postwar affluence while also managing their bodies for optimal health? Over the next three decades, health experts and the American population at large struggled to reconcile the physical needs of their bodies with an environment that had made them largely irrelevant. The solution to this problem was the invention of exercise.

It's tempting to view the ascendance of fitness culture as an inevitable process, the natural result of an increasingly prosperous society seeking methods to compensate for decreased physical activity in daily life. But thinking of exercise as a foregone conclusion would be a mistake. The acceptance of exercise was a gradual process and one that met with tremendous opposition. Although midcentury Americans worried about the long-term consequences—both physical and mental—of their comfortable existence, it was unclear that dedicated physical activity could solve the problem. For the better part of two decades, questions about the necessity of exercise, the types of suitable activities, the appropriate level of intensity, and exercise's effectiveness were the subject of heated discussion. Compounding this widespread confusion was the cultural perception that exercise was not something that upstanding middle-class men engaged in, nor was it believed to be useful in helping women lose weight. And science offered little insight—some physicians readily admitted ignorance, while others labeled exercise dangerous.

Understanding the historical underpinnings of exercise culture sheds light on our current beliefs about fitness and its role in our lives, many of which have emerged only recently. This book decouples the recent twinning of diet and exercise, traces the medical profession's reluctant acceptance of exercise, documents that baby boomers were not the first exercising generation, and investigates how, as fitness activities became more intense and physically demanding over time, they also became more closely linked to notions of virtue, moral purity, and power. In the last case in particular, the knowledge that these ideas are manufactured gives us the power to debunk them as essential truths.

This book begins in the 1950s, a time of exceptional cultural change. The two-decade period following the end of World War II brought a return to normalcy and an emphasis on domestic life; it also brought prosperity and sweeping technological innovations to a rapidly expanding middle class. This period witnessed the mass exodus of Americans from urban areas to newly developed suburbs. It is not a coincidence that concerns about body weight and decreasing physical activity emerged at the same time that single-family suburban homes were becoming the preference among most Americans. Decentralized home construction led to immense changes in how people lived in their homes, went to school and work, purchased groceries, and used their leisure time. The fact that the new suburban lifestyle was changing their bodies was readily apparent to Americans of the era. Though they rarely expressed these changes as "suburbanization"—preferring phrases such as "our modern way of life"—parents, government officials, and physicians worried that the nation's citizens were becoming both less fit and heavier because of subtle environmental changes that, as an ensemble, decreased physical activity and encouraged sedentary recreation.[4] In 1952, the National Institutes of Health declared obesity the nation's number-one nutritional problem.[5] A year later, a research study revealed that American children were less fit than their European counterparts.[6] Americans viewed such pronouncements as proof that school buses, widespread car ownership, television (not necessarily a part of suburban life, but often associated with it), and central heating had removed much of the physical activity from daily life. Even new one-story ranch houses—which lacked exercise-inducing stairs—were cited as evidence that life had become too easy.

The suburban migration of the mid-twentieth century is one of the most studied phenomena in American history, yet surprisingly, no scholar has considered its effects on the bodies of the first generation of suburbanites.[7] Today, we know that the physical environment plays a significant role in encouraging (or discouraging) physical activity. Walkable neighborhoods, park and trail proximity, and safe public spaces are crucial elements in making movement part of one's daily routine. Research has linked suburban and exurban lifestyles with decreased physical activity, higher body weights, and a greater likelihood of obesity and hypertension.[8] An analysis of more than 200,000 adults by the National Center for Smart Growth, for example, revealed that people living in regions with the highest "sprawl index" were more likely to have a higher body mass index, weight, blood pressure, and risk of obesity.[9] Unfortunately, similar studies don't exist for the postwar era; however, we can trace the physical changes associated with suburbanization through the comments and publications of midcentury Americans, the rising rates of "affluenza"-related conditions such as coronary heart disease, nationwide weight gain, and growing interest in fitness.[10]

Although this book takes the 1950s as its point of departure, readers should not assume that American physical culture began then. Americans have been profoundly interested in physical development and the cultivation of health since colonial times. The period around the turn of the twentieth century has been particularly well documented by historians. Between 1880 and 1920, figures such as domestic adviser Catharine Beecher; Dudley Sargent, athletic director at Harvard; Luther Gulick, founder of the YMCA; strongman Eugen Sandow; and President Theodore Roosevelt played crucial roles in popularizing the active life for men and women. At the time, physical activity was often undertaken in service of a higher goal. The muscular Christianity movement, as well as the institutional church-synagogue movement, espoused the notion that physical activity and the perfection of the body could bring a believer closer to God. For men of the upper classes, such as Teddy Roosevelt, physical activity was an expression of dominance and manliness that could rejuvenate "overcivilized" bodies whose poor physical state threatened the continued existence of the "white race."[11]

In the 1920s and beyond, fitness pursuits took a decidedly more self-centered, individual turn. Rather than the betterment of one's morals, religion, or race, physical development became important for its ability to help one fit in and advance in life. Historian Warren Susman famously noted that it was about this time that the idea of "personality" displaced "character" as a foundational quality in the construction of the self. The first decades of the twentieth century, Susman believed, witnessed the birth of a new kind of personal identity derived from an intense search for self-fulfillment and one's own uniqueness, complemented by a need to make oneself appealing to others. Values that had traditionally been correlated with character, such as duty, work, citizenship, and honor, began to play a diminished role in one's conception of self and became less useful in the transaction of modern life.[12] In an increasingly impersonal, urban world, self-presentation became an art.

This transition can be seen in the 1920s and 1930s in the world of physical culture. Thanks to the efforts of fitness entrepreneurs Bernarr MacFadden and Charles Atlas; a cohort of bodybuilders and fitness enthusiasts that included Earle Liederman, Joe Bonomo, Sig Klein, Jack La Lanne, and Vic Tanny; and the film exploits of Douglas Fairbanks and Johnny Weissmuller, a physical culture founded on personal development and magnetism began to form. MacFadden, Atlas, Tanny, and La Lanne all espoused the belief that a regular regimen of physical activity could improve one's ability to find employment, be successful, attract a partner, and enjoy life. The timing of these efforts is noteworthy. Although many of their names are familiar, these men have often been viewed as singular figures, not associated with any larger movement. And it's often assumed that the Depression and World War II ended the interest in fitness, which would not emerge again until the 1970s. But this is far from the case. La Lanne and Tanny made their first forays into the fitness business in the 1930s; the trade in cabinet cards featuring bodybuilders—many of whom operated their own gyms—increased awareness of the muscular physique; and the popularity of MacFadden's sanatoria and his magazine *Physical Culture* and Atlas's Dynamic Tension course, attest to the persistence of fitness culture, even in trying times. In fact, according to Atlas's business partner Charles Roman, unemployed men were actually good for business because they had more time for exercise: "Also they figure maybe the reason they are out of work is because they lack physical power. We always do well in hard times in this business."[13] While wartime mobilization certainly impacted the consumer health market—athletic club rosters, for example, were depleted during the war, causing many clubs to close—the need for physically powerful soldiers brought attention to exercise and resulted in Hale America, a national fitness drive.[14]

In the postwar period, federal exercise promotion efforts; television exercise shows; exercise books, records, and gadgets; workplace fitness programs; and the influence of preventive health research all spurred Americans to get moving (or at least to wonder whether they should) in the 1950s and 1960s. Scholarship as well as popular thinking typically point to the

1970s as the beginning of the American fitness "craze," but this historical sketch and the chapters that follow delineate a continuum in Americans' interest in and practice of exercise throughout the twentieth century. This contrasts greatly with the cycles of boom and bust that have traditionally been associated with the history of physical culture.[15]

One likely explanation for this piecemeal view of physical culture history is the difficulty of conducting historical research in a field that often leaves little in the way of a paper trail. Documents related to consumer health quickly become obsolete with new scientific findings (libraries, for example, often see no reason to keep dated health publications), fitness businesses rarely preserve their records (especially during periods of financial upheaval), and fitness associations, including those that are successful and long-lived, often fail to recognize the historical value of their archival collections. Even other scholars have tended to discount the historical value of exercise- and health-related research.[16] It's logical, then, that historical treatments of physical culture have focused on periods of intense fervor that provided significant documentation. The difficulty of locating materials should not be taken as proof of a lack of interest in the body or its maintenance, however.

Today when we think about exercise, lifting weights at the gym, fitness classes, jogging, and yoga are likely to come to mind. Although there are certainly countless pursuits one can undertake in the name of physical exertion, the circumscription of exercise as a handful of specialized, noncompetitive, individual activities conducted outside of one's daily routine, usually involving distinctive clothing and footwear and performed at a dedicated location, has narrowed the way we think about exercise and increased the lengths we believe we have to go to engage in it. In the 1950s, the President's Council on Youth Fitness stated that "there were no minor sports." Fishing, camping, and bowling were considered just as fitness enhancing as bicycling, baseball, and calisthenics. That the council typically discussed the acquisition of fitness through sports rather than exercise spoke to the latter's novelty. In the past, getting exercise was usually the by-product of playing a game or a sport, not something one engaged in simply for the sake of self-development. Nor were fitness activities imagined as necessarily labor intensive or sweat inducing. Getting a massage, sitting in a steam room, taking a stretching class, and engaging in vigorous calisthenics—all activities done in the name of fitness—were viewed as equally beneficial, demonstrating the breadth of the fitness concept at midcentury. The lack of a working definition of fitness during the 1950s and 1960s allowed exercisers the freedom to make their own choices regarding physical activity but at the same time made it difficult for physicians to make recommendations for their patients. Not until 1968, when physician Kenneth Cooper's book *Aerobics* explained the "training effect" in lay terms, would most Americans agree on the factors that constituted fitness.[17]

There is tremendous fluidity in the way fitness has been defined through the decades. Even today, physical educators, health experts, and sports authorities define the term differently.[18] When Cooper defined fitness in terms of cardiovascular function and launched the jogging movement, his recommendations were decidedly modest—around three hours of exercise per week for most ability levels. He never imagined that this amount of exercise would soon be seen as a trifle by many fitness buffs. It didn't take long for "jogging" to become "running" by the 1970s, for marathon participation to surge, and for exercise to be accompanied by profound exhaustion. Cooper refuted the idea that becoming healthy required endurance sports and heavy perspiration, observing, "If you run more than 15 miles a week you're running for something other than cardiovascular fitness."[19]

That "something" illustrates that fitness had become more than just a matter of health maintenance. Workplace fitness initiatives associated paid labor with fitness (along with the ability to make time for it all), and the lifestyle-changing regularity of a jogging habit helped bring a new sense of moralism to exercise culture toward the end of the 1960s. Maintaining a regular workout routine soon became a demonstration of one's interior mettle. And if being an exerciser somehow made you a better person, it followed that people who didn't work out (or at least looked like they didn't) were lazy, unmotivated, and undisciplined.

For all the physical benefits it provides, exercise should not be viewed as an unassailable good. A certain measure of physical activity is necessary for one's well-being, but the value judgments, associations, and moralisms that have become a part of fitness culture complicate the practice of exercise. Ideas about the kind of people who exercise, what exercising bodies should look like, and the inner values supposedly reflected by fit (read thin) bodies play a role in getting us to the gym (or keeping us away). As a health practice, exercise is complicit in the culture of medicalization that holds that all health-seeking behaviors are meritorious. In the first fifty years of the twentieth century, vaccinations, antibiotics, and modern medicine cultivated a culture in which physicians bore the responsibility for their patients' health. With the recognition of modern disease risk factors such as tobacco use, poor dietary habits, and a sedentary lifestyle, the responsibility for good health was returned to the individual. In fact, in the modern era, health is often seen as a personal accomplishment.[20]

As Jonathan Metzl explains in *Against Health: How Health Became the New Morality*, when we castigate someone for smoking, what we really mean is: "you are a bad person because you smoke."[21] In fitness culture, similar judgments occur. Job candidates, for example, are often advised to mention their fitness interests during interviews because running and other active pursuits are considered marks of discipline and achievement—desirable characteristics in an employee. But it's interesting to note how recently our belief that exercise reflects self-mastery came into existence. In the 1950s, there was no virtue to be gained from strenuous exercise. In fact, men who were preoccupied with their bodies were the objects of suspicion and derision. By the late 1960s, however, the media's frequent coverage of exercising chief executives and company gyms began to create an image of the exerciser as a highly competent, driven individual who stretched the limits of the workday to make time for exercise, which was not a pleasurable hobby but a serious avocation crucial to keeping the employee healthy for work. The linkages between exercise and moral superiority were solidified through the 1970s and 1980s. Many new joggers made no bones about the fact that their exercise routines made them better people than their nonexercising neighbors, and the trend toward longer distances only increased this effect. In the following decade, the emphasis on muscles meant that the evidence of one's workout routine was on display, even outside the gym. In short, the fit body had become a new form of physical capital.

Understanding the cultural baggage we have attached to the practice of exercise is critical if the goal is to make exercising for health a priority for *all* Americans. "Health is a term replete with value judgments, hierarchies, and blind assumptions that speak as much about power and privilege as they do about well-being," Metzl notes in *Against Health*.[22] As the following pages document, exercise was typically a pastime of the white middle and upper classes. Disposable time, disposable income, and access to health information were all necessary factors in teaching twentieth-century Americans to make exercise a habit. As fitness culture evolved, the media increasingly described it as a preoccupation of wealthy white achievers. The men's cardiac crisis of the 1950s—the spike in heart attacks that sparked middle-class interest in exercising for health—was portrayed as a problem of the privileged. Once exercise was seen as the solution to health and figure problems in the 1960s, it was similarly depicted as a leisure activity of the elite. In a 1968 account of the exercise routines of Washington politicians and government officials and their wives, the *New York Times* made it clear that physical culture was no longer the province of the immigrant strongman: "In the basement of the fashionable home of Mrs. E. Rudolph Carter, the wife of a State Department official, Mrs. Damon leads a growing list of young social types in toning up exercises to music. She shouts out directions in English and French for her exacting routines—a combination of Swedish gym and ballet exercises—that she originally worked up for Queen Sirikit of Thailand when Mr. Damon was stationed in Bangkok."[23] With its numerous linkages to high culture, this anecdote illustrates that exercise had risen in status.

As a technique to exorcise the perils of consumption, exercise promotion efforts were rarely directed toward those who had yet to benefit from the nation's culture of abundance. Exercise was imagined to be a replacement for the physical activity that had been lost to sedentary, "desk-bound" work; the nation's lower classes were largely assumed to be engaged in work that had some measure of physicality. In the 1962 CBS documentary *The Fat American*, Harvard nutritionist Jean Mayer informed journalist Harry Reasoner, "We are rapidly getting to the point where the only people who exercise in an organization are the chairman of the board and the janitor. The chairman because he can afford to, the janitor because he has to."[24]

This presumption typically meant that Americans of color were excluded from exercise awareness campaigns, both federal and commercial. This is reflected in the scant reporting on exercise in the African American media. Although exercise for weight loss was occasionally covered in articles for female readers, black media outlets did not begin to cover exercise as part of a healthy lifestyle until the 1970s, when jogging expanded in popularity, and even then, it received less attention than in other publications. This historical omission is likely responsible, at least in part, for contemporary low rates of exercise participation among people of color.[25] In a recent survey on exercise, an African American participant explained, "I feel that my culture often views physical activity as an unaffordable luxury," illustrating the longevity of class associations that grew in tandem with fitness culture.[26]

During the 1950s and 1960s, exercise underwent an image makeover as fitness entrepreneurs rehabilitated the public's perception of fitness pursuits, displacing dark, smelly gyms and compulsory physical education classes with modern, luxurious-feeling health clubs and an emphasis on fun. Unfortunately, this cultural realignment heightened the racial and class differences in the types of activities people were supposed to engage in. For Americans outside the middle class, both black and white, physical activity was more likely to occur within the context of organized sports than fitness for health. And although opportunities to pursue physical development for its own sake existed in the black community, such as in historically black YMCAs, sports offered the possibility of victory and, for the athletically gifted, a path to potential financial success.

Cultural perceptions about the value of exercise also play a role in our health choices. An awareness of the long-lasting effects of these historical biases can help make exercise more accessible to everyone and resolve persistent health disparities. It's not clear, however, that awareness of the benefits of exercise or even the practice of a regular fitness routine will be enough to mitigate the effects of modern American lifestyles, even among the privileged. Setting aside time for exercise is difficult, despite the desire to do so. Work schedules, long commutes, and the demands of family life limit the time available for exercise, especially as we define the term now. Leisure time today often translates to (sedentary) screen time. And too often we fall victim to enjoinders to overconsume, especially high-calorie, unhealthy foods whose prices are kept artificially low by federal agricultural subsidies, undermining the government's exercise promotion efforts.[27] Although fitness culture is a significant aspect of American popular culture, reversing the effects of our modern way of life continues to be a challenge.

Looking at exercise culture through the decades illustrates how Americans of an earlier era understood their bodies, their health, and their duties as citizens. Exercise books and records, television shows, and related advertising often functioned as a form of cultural critique. In their desire for healthier, higher-functioning bodies, Americans often expressed a longing for a more physically demanding time—one that (they imagined) shaped physique as much as character. The softer, postwar bodies that cold warriors derided were proof that the nation's new affluence was not always considered a boon. The realization that a changing environment had also changed bodies was a frightening one.

This book's first chapter, based on research at the National Archives, explores the history of the President's Council on Youth Fitness (PCYF), established under Eisenhower in response to physical fitness tests that revealed American children were weaker than their European counterparts. Though largely forgotten today, the PCYF, predecessor of the current President's Council on Physical Fitness, Sports, and Nutrition conducted an intense public information campaign to raise awareness of "total fitness," seeking to encourage not only physical fitness but also "mental, moral, emotional, social and cultural fitness." This multifocal mission concealed the council's true aims of curbing juvenile delinquency, offsetting the dangerous effects of postwar affluence, and creating a generation of soldiers who could resist communist brainwashing. Though the council's campaign to make personal physical fitness the goal of every American child was ultimately unsuccessful, those efforts laid the groundwork for a new fitness industry in the years to come.

A pair of subsequent chapters investigates gender differences in commercial exercise promotion in the midcentury period. Chapter 2 explores the new culture of thinness and weight reduction for women in the late 1950s and 1960s, using research from women's magazines and exercise books, records, and television shows. The media of that era informed wives that maintaining an attractive figure was a crucial part of the marriage bargain. Early fitness instructors warned women that without careful attention to their figures, their husbands might lose interest. New television exercise shows took to the airwaves to instruct suburban housewives how to tone and shape their bodies and, in doing so, constructed the practice of exercise as both a daily chore and a welcome break from household drudgery. Jack La Lanne and his colleagues enthusiastically promoted exercise as the answer to what Betty Friedan had termed "the problem with no name," and the list of benefits exercise was said to bestow gradually expanded to include happiness, sexual desirability, and other personality-enhancing qualities.

While women's exercise was solely for beautification, exercise for men was a matter of life and death. Despite long-held beliefs about the sense of virtue derived from a personal exercise routine, middle-class men of the mid-twentieth century initially found few reasons to take up exercise. It took the cardiac crisis—a dramatic escalation in the number of heart attacks among men and the cultural panic surrounding it—to generate interest in exercise as a preventive health measure. This attention to men's health gave physicians a platform to speak about preventive health care (giving rise to the new field of executive health and a spate of heart attack prevention manuals), and it provided ample opportunity for doctors to prescribe exercise—thereby increasing its cultural acceptance—but physicians offered relatively little in the way of specific advice. Instead, as "guardians of family health," wives were instructed to manage their husbands' diets, schedule checkups, and relieve stress. This increased women's power within the household, but it also encouraged their husbands to abdicate responsibility for their own health.

Chapter 4 explores the origins of jogging and the motivations that propelled exercisers into the streets in the 1960s and 1970s. The publication of two books on jogging in the late 1960s capitalized on more than a decade of exercise promotion that had, as yet, found no real outlet. Together, Bill Bowerman's *Jogging* and Ken Cooper's *Aerobics* promoted an easygoing, progressive approach to exercise that defined success in terms of consistency and heart health, rather than wins and losses. Jogging was "discovered" over the course of the decade by two distinct groups. Originally marketed as a technique to maintain health, jogging found its first group of adherents among a decidedly middle-aged population. A second, younger group, motivated by environmental and spiritual concerns, adopted jogging later in the decade for its own, often political and psychological, purposes. As it found nationwide appeal, jogging united exercisers across the political spectrum: for conservative politicians, regular exercise was a means to decrease health care costs and demonstrate concern for the pocketbooks of their fellow citizens; for seekers of alternative health care, jogging represented a new kind of self-care. Although they took to tracks and trails with different aims, these disparate groups joined forces to make fitness a mass movement.

The final chapter examines the history of the health club in the United States, with a focus on the 1980s. Health clubs grew in both number and membership over the course of the decade, thanks to the invention of Nautilus equipment, the advent of aerobics in gyms, and the muscular aesthetic, creating a new kind of community space, albeit a privatized one. The patriotic rhetoric of toughness that President Ronald Reagan brought to office injected exercise culture with a new intensity that, exercisers believed, gave them a competitive edge in both personal and professional life. Taken together, these changes reinvigorated the sense of virtue exercisers achieved by working out; in the 1980s, a fit body was a morally correct body. But even as working out became increasingly demanding, it created new opportunities for friendship, romance, and community. The chapter ends with a discussion of health clubs as a new kind of "third place," drawing on historical examples of straight and gay social life, including a discussion of AIDS and weight lifting, and arguing that health clubs provide valuable sites of social interaction.

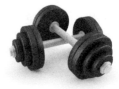

I

Much like the slow-burning detonation cord in old cartoons, the news that American children were unfit traveled slowly through the halls of Washington before it exploded in political crisis. In 1953, physician Hans Kraus and exercise enthusiast Ruth P. Hirschland traveled to Austria and Italy, where they administered a battery of fitness tests designed by Kraus and his colleague, Dr. Sonja Weber, to children aged six to nineteen to investigate the causes of backaches in adults. The Kraus-Weber tests were composed of a number of exercises to measure what the researchers had deemed "minimum fitness levels": toe touching to measure hamstring flexibility, sit-ups and leg lifts to measure abdominal strength, and prone leg and torso lifts to measure back strength. Kraus and Hirschland had previously examined several groups of American children, and their European tests were conducted only for purposes of comparison. Expecting to find similar results between the two groups, they were astonished to find major differences: while 56 percent of the American children had failed the tests, only 8 percent of the European children had.[1]

Kraus and Hirschland attributed the high rate of failure among the American children to the fact that "European children do not have the benefit of a highly mechanized society; they do not use cars, school buses, elevators or any other labor-saving devices. They must walk everywhere.

Their recreation is largely based on the active use of their own bodies." Their three-page report argued for expanded physical fitness programs and testing for children, especially younger ones, and warned that "insufficient exercise may cause the dropping of muscle efficiency levels below that necessary for daily living."[2]

Unlike most academic articles, Kraus and Hirschland's work did not go unnoticed. In fact, within a few months, word of the study had reached the ears of the president, and newspapers and magazines across the United States were reporting that American children were unfit, sparking a national conversation about fitness. *Cosmopolitan* asked, "Are We and Our Children Getting Too Soft?" *Ladies' Home Journal* wondered, "How Fit Are Our Children?" and *Newsweek* explained in a lengthy article "Why the President Is Worried about Our Fitness."[3] Set against profound anxieties about postwar abundance, baby boom child rearing, and the Cold War, the Kraus-Hirschland study seemed to offer concrete proof that there *was* a problem with America's children and suggested that if their bodies could be reformed, so could they.

President Eisenhower reacted swiftly to news of the study's results by establishing the President's Council on Youth Fitness (PCYF). During its five-year existence, the now largely forgotten council conducted an intensive public information campaign to raise awareness of fitness. From 1956 to 1960, the PCYF maintained a constant media presence that reminded parents and youth alike that it was their civic duty to get their bodies—and their minds—in shape. Although most Americans and many scholars cite the Kennedy administration's President's Council on Physical Fitness as the first national fitness campaign, it was in fact the PCYF that brought the concept of personal fitness to national attention.[4] In so doing, the council helped broaden consumer interest in exercise and paved the way for a dramatic expansion of the commercial fitness industry in the 1960s. As a governmental agency created at the height of the Cold War, however, the council embedded its physical fitness message within a more complex rhetoric of reform that envisioned children as future parents, citizens, and soldiers whose moral, mental, and physical capabilities were key to maintaining the superiority of the nation both at home and abroad.

Although a study on physical fitness had precipitated the PCYF's establishment, those involved in setting it up quickly expanded its mission to include the well-being of American children in all areas. Council organizers interpreted *fitness*—a word that, in the 1950s, did not automatically connote physical condition—as fitness in all possible senses. The first youth fitness conference, held at the U.S. Naval Academy in Annapolis in 1956, defined *fitness* as an idea that "encompasses the total person—spiritual, mental, emotional, social, cultural as well as the physical."[5] The mission of "total fitness" allowed the PCYF to address numerous postwar anxieties with its campaign: exercise would be one part of a total plan designed to resolve the juvenile delinquency crisis; improve both physical and mental aptitude for military service; counteract the perceived detrimental effects of a new, higher standard of living; and help educate young Americans about the duties of citizenship in a democracy.

President Eisenhower had first been alerted to the Kraus-Hirschland study by Pennsylvania senator James H. Duff. Duff had originally been contacted by constituent John B. Kelly, a prominent Philadelphian, a sculling champion, and the father of Princess Grace, who had organized the short-lived World War II fitness drive called Hale America. Highlighting a theme that would recur during discussions about national fitness, Duff expressed concern that the muscular strength that had made westward expansion possible was now in jeopardy. "Here we are only a few generations removed from the frontier and one of the most serious problems facing us now is the physical deterioration of our youth," he wrote to Eisenhower.[6] As Duff and Kelly saw the situation, forceful, mighty bodies were an integral part of the nation's heritage, and their potential loss could mean the end of the American empire.

The Kraus-Weber tests crystallized a number of fears regarding American bodies. The prosperous years of the postwar economic boom had created a rapidly growing middle class that avidly purchased suburban homes, automobiles, and "push-button gadgets."[7] But as welcome as these goods were, they also sparked worries that luxury was corrosive, leading to physical laziness and mental sloth. Many of the lifestyle changes cited in Kraus and Hirschland's article were true: suburban children now rode buses to school rather than walked, television occupied a large portion of Americans' leisure hours, and the increased automation of factories and the expansion of the service industry called for less physical movement at work. Simply put, physical abilities were less important in this new landscape. These changes conflicted with closely held ideas about a shared national past and the physical characteristics necessary for productive citizenship, however. The American body was a fit body, poised to take action and able to endure hardship, a visible symbol of physical power. It had been instrumental in conquering the West, winning two world wars, and establishing a strong economy on the backs of able workers. New Deal–era artwork of the 1930s, for example, portrayed sculpted, muscular bodies in the service of national memory. Depression-era murals from the Federal Art Project relied heavily on agricultural and labor themes, featuring muscular workers toiling for the nation.[8] Americans imagined that their forebears used these strong bodies to forge a nation, and they relied on such depictions in artwork to find strength in the midst of the Depression. Christina Jarvis's analysis of World War II–era images—Uncle Sam and Rosie the Riveter, folk heroes Paul Bunyan and John Henry, combat-themed advertising, and superhero imagery—similarly illustrates how physical hardiness was an integral part of the national identity, providing reassurance during trying times.[9] The idea that Americans were a muscular people and, by extension, fit and strong was buttressed by the belief that Americans had access to the best health care system in the world and enjoyed a superior diet that only a land of plenty could provide.[10] The notion, then, that Americans were becoming unfit, soft, weak, or flabby—adjectives the news media employed in the wake of the fitness report—represented nothing less than the destruction of a national myth.

More specifically, news of the fitness report was troubling because it portended a weak military force. The results of the Kraus-Weber tests were viewed as both an explanation of past problems in military staffing and evidence that such issues would continue. Because physical abilities were seen as instrumental to winning the Cold War, it was imperative that a solution be found to the fitness problem. Figures from World War I, World War II, and the Korean War indicated that American draftees were failing their induction physicals at dramatic rates. Widespread media coverage suggested that soon there wouldn't be enough fit men to maintain an ad-

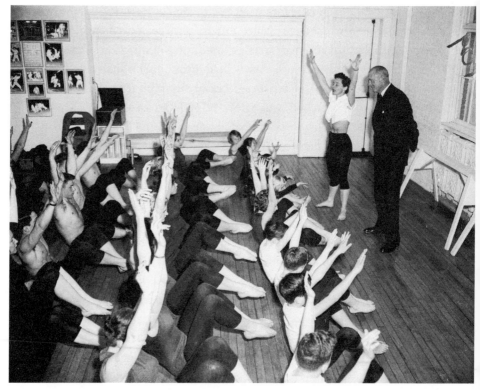

Former Olympian John B. Kelly observes Bonnie Prudden (formerly Ruth Hirschland) conducting a class at her school, the Institute for Physical Fitness, in White Plains, New York. Kelly was responsible for bringing Prudden and Hans Kraus's study of children's fitness to national attention. (© Bettman/Corbis)

equate military. Moreover, soldiers already in the armed forces were seen as increasingly ill equipped to serve. Anecdotal reports abounded that men were not as tough as they used to be. John Kelly attributed the nation's military softness to a higher standard of living during the formative years: "I've often heard combat veterans say that, man for man, the Japanese infantryman of World War II was a much tougher soldier than his American counterpart. Because of his rugged childhood, he could march farther and endure more privations."[11] Just as the launching of *Sputnik* jump-started a host of science and math initiatives in schools, the Kraus-Hirschland report began a national conversation about fitness and the American way of life that began in 1953 and continued in the media, the political sphere, and the home throughout the decade, raising important questions about human bodies and how to maintain them in the context of postwar abundance.

Establishing the Council

It's not surprising that national fitness efforts were first directed toward children. Between 1946 and 1964, 78 million Americans were born, leading to an unprecedented population boom. During the decade of the 1950s, births hovered at around 4 million a year—a U.S. record.[12] As this group transitioned into adolescence, a distinct teen culture emerged with its own music, fashion, dance, and language. At the same time, these increasingly independent adolescents, who often had their own cars and pocket money, were targeted by a plethora of new teen-directed magazines, films, comic books, television programs, and advertising. The sheer number of young adults, combined with decreasing parental influence and reports of delinquent behavior, created the perception of "a storm of criminality [that] was rumbling across the nation."[13] Child development experts, parents, politicians, and law enforcement officials seemed to agree that adolescents had become more prone to commit crimes. As one sociologist commented, "Rowdiness in and out of school, abuse of driving privileges, joy-riding, thefts, excessive drinking, vandalism and sexual misconduct are among the principal forms of disapproved acts seemingly becoming more frequent among teenagers from 'better' backgrounds."[14]

The belief that a generation of young Americans was out of control led Congress to take action. The Senate Judiciary Subcommittee on Juvenile Delinquency, chaired by Estes Kefauver, blamed comics, television, and the cinema for the increase in crimes, keeping the topic in the news as it held hearings in a number of American cities through the 1950s.[15] While purportedly investigating the causes of poor behavior among teens, these hearings—and the coverage of them—added to the perception that teenagers across the country were running wild. These were the first televised governmental hearings of any kind, and according to one estimate, 86 percent of American television sets were tuned in when they aired.[16] In addition, Hollywood took advantage of the salacious topic to turn out a spate of delinquency films—with titles such as *Rebel without a Cause, Blackboard Jungle, Teen-Age Crime Wave, Crime in the Streets,* and *The Delinquents*—perpetuating the notion of teens gone wild.[17]

Although juvenile delinquency had been a newsworthy topic since the 1940s, it reached a peak between 1953 and 1956—the same time fitness was identified as a problem.[18] Early planning documents and media reports about the PCYF indicate that organizers considered improving physical fitness a desirable goal because it could also help curtail delinquent behavior. Physical fitness programs could occupy leisure hours, channel excess energy, and "improve" the character of youth through fitness activities, especially organized competitive sports. Eisenhower explained in a letter: "At the suggestion of one of my friends, I am trying to bring together a number of outstanding sports figures. The aim of the meeting is to see what we can do about combatting juvenile delinquency and substituting an increasing interest in sports among young people."[19] Media coverage emphasized the delinquency connection, and the public also believed that a national fitness program would reduce juvenile delinquency. In a poll of sports figures and celebrities, more than half mentioned decreased delinquency as a benefit of children's exercising.[20] Eisenhower assigned Vice President Richard Nixon to oversee the fitness initiative, which Nixon described as having the "dual purpose of increasing the physical fitness of our youth through sports participation, as well as developing a powerful weapon against juvenile delinquency."[21]

References to juvenile delinquency began to diminish quickly, however, as the council set about its work. Presidential aide Bob King warned early in the organizing process that overtly promoting fitness as an antidelinquency measure would discourage some children from participating in fitness programs.[22] And just two weeks before the first youth fitness conference, President Eisenhower similarly indicated that any successful program to curb delinquency would have to obscure its intention to do so. Responding to a proposal by a navy official, Eisenhower asserted that the program "should contain no hint that it is for the purpose of curbing juvenile delinquency. I really believe the words 'juvenile delinquency' are doing as much as any other that I can think of to defeat our purposes in this regard." Instead, he suggested a focus on "something positive; namely, the sane, healthy development of our children morally, intellectually and physically."[23] Thus, messages that linked delinquency with fitness were deliberately downplayed in favor of a more positive spin on the benefits of fitness and sports. This trend was also encouraged by the gradual decline of the delinquency hysteria, which faded as fear of teenage rebellion gave way to acceptance of the new teen subculture. Although overt references to juvenile delinquency disappeared from council literature, the association between fitness and the development of good behavior and character did not.[24] PCYF staff remained intensely interested in the mental and physical development of youth, but the framework that shaped these twin goals shifted away from delinquency to two broader concerns, both of which allowed council organizers to continue their interest in creating upstanding youth, albeit within a different context.

The effect of the postwar economic boom and the proliferation of consumer goods on the national character and American bodies was just as troublesome a topic as delinquency. Fitness proponents were worried that a higher living standard was weakening Americans both physically and mentally. A life of ease simply could not create the same kind of citizens that hardship had. As *Cosmopolitan* observed, "The handwriting isn't on the wall. It is in the slack muscles, bulging stomachs and growing passivity of American men, women, and children."[25] Second, the recently ended Korean War, Cold War tensions, and worry about how to prepare future generations of soldiers loomed large in the minds of PCYF organizers. Both these issues (along with juvenile delinquency) involved physical as well as mental or moral components, explaining the council's preference for a policy of "total fitness" rather than one focused solely on the physical. It wasn't enough to develop the bodies of American children; their minds also required training for good citizenship and proper behavior.

Throughout 1954, the press continued to discuss American children and their bodies, keeping the topic of youth fitness in the news. Magazines and newspapers lamented the lack of physical fitness education in schools, debated the merits of competitive sports (which focused on the athletically gifted) versus physical training for all children, speculated about the impact of postwar prosperity on American bodies, and complained about unfit soldiers who were too "soft" to defend the county.

Hans Kraus and Bonnie Prudden (formerly Ruth Hirschland, who was now using her nickname and maiden name after a divorce) also kept fitness in the news with frequent comments in the popular press and new versions of their material in the professional realm.[26] It wasn't until 1955, however, that the White House took formal action. During the summer, the administration organized two luncheons that included professional athletes, Kraus and Prudden, government officials, and executives from nonprofit organizations associated with children, recreation, and health.[27] These meetings resulted in plans for a two-day conference on youth fitness in September at Lowry Air Force Base in Colorado, where Vice President Nixon would oversee the proceedings.[28] But when President Eisenhower suffered a heart attack on September 23, 1955, the conference was postponed until June 1956.[29] Meanwhile, the media continued to keep fitness in the public eye.

The rescheduled conference, held at the U.S. Naval Academy, was attended by 149 educators; health, youth, and sports association presidents; military officers; and media organization heads. Invitees, who traveled to Maryland at their own expense, included Roy Larsen, editor of Time; Ralph Hardy of CBS; Thomas Velota of ABC; Harry Wismer of Mutual Broadcasting; Leo Peterson, sports editor of United Press; and Sidney James, editor of Sports Illustrated. Their participation ensured that the meeting would attract publicity.

The conference resulted in the issuing of Executive Order 10673, which established the PCYF and the President's Citizens Advisory Committee on the Fitness of American Youth (PCAC), a group of prominent Americans that would advise the council as well as promote its goals.[30] Shane MacCarthy, an Irish-born lawyer, former CIA employee, and father of five sons, was named executive director of the council.[31] Appointees to the PCAC were primarily professionals from various national sports, youth, and recreation associations; they volunteered their time, paid their own expenses to attend meetings, and served one-year terms. The chair of the advisory committee, though not necessarily based in Washington, played a larger role in PCYF affairs, acting as a deputy to MacCarthy.

During the five years MacCarthy led the PCYF, it held annual conferences; sponsored an annual national Youth Fitness Week; published nu-

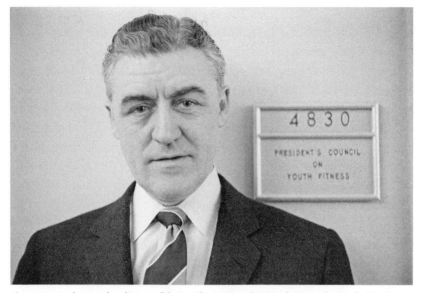

Shane MacCarthy served as director of the President's Council on Youth Fitness during the Eisenhower administration. Although MacCarthy's efforts to make total fitness the goal of every American child failed, the PCYF was unintentionally responsible for making fitness a national buzzword and launching a nascent industry. (Photograph by Douglas Jones, Look Magazine Photograph Collection, Prints and Photographs Division, Library of Congress, LC Job 57-7062-J-11)

merous reports, brochures, and posters; produced radio spots and television commercials; and, above all, encouraged fitness initiatives through its work with corporations, national and local nonprofit organizations, and state and local governments. Essentially, the PCYF was a public relations firm for the notion of fitness. It did not directly sponsor any physical fitness activities, clinics, or instructor training. It did not conduct or sponsor scientific research. Instead, council staff worked to get others excited about improving the nation's fitness.

According to MacCarthy, the PCYF's role was to be "a catalyst, a stimulator, a coordinator, a persuader, an urger, an idea-dropper, a direction-pointer."[32] MacCarthy was a tireless fitness promoter who appeared on countless national and local radio broadcasts and television shows and wrote editorials for both mainstream and specialty media. He logged hundreds of thousands of miles during his tenure, making speeches and public appearances. One PCYF newsletter quipped that he was second only to

Secretary of State John Foster Dulles in the number of air miles he traveled.[33] Deputy director Ott Romney and other staff members also made
numerous personal appearances.[34] PCAC members were encouraged to
undertake promotional efforts similar to MacCarthy's, and many of them,
especially the PCAC chair, did so with enthusiasm. MacCarthy was a true
believer who ranked the fitness campaign on the same level of importance
as Jonas Salk's polio vaccine or the space race. Given his limited budget
and staff, MacCarthy's role in the promotion of physical fitness in the
1950s cannot be overstated; that *fitness* became such a buzzword during
the decade was due in large part to his efforts.

PROMOTING FITNESS

One of the PCYF's first challenges was to decide what *American* fitness was.
As news of the council's establishment made its way through the media,
letters from around the country arrived at PCYF headquarters warning that
any kind of standardized physical fitness program would be un-American.
For many, such programs conjured up images of Nazi Germany or the
Soviet Union. In an editorial, the *Pittsburgh Post* admitted that fitness was
tantamount to "national survival" but wondered how it could be accom-
plished in a democratic nation. "The problem is to motivate a peace-loving
and democratic people to achieve fitness without mass regimentation—as
some nations do—and above all, to prove that it can be attained in a society where individual freedom is cherished. . . . We hope, however, that
[Eisenhower] will avoid anything resembling Hitler's 'Strength through
Joy' program. Nor would we relish the sight of acres of American youths
assembled à la Moscow, for mass calisthenics."[35] John Kelly, originally
alarmed by the Kraus-Hirschland study, was equally critical of any kind of
mandatory national program. "Totalitarians have an easy way to cope with
body, mind, spirit," he pointed out. "Order the boys and girls to do their
sitting-up exercises. Order them into the lab to work out a little rocketry.
Order them to read Marx and salute Lenin's tomb. Around the democra-
cies, we have a more complicated view. We urge the boys and girls to do
what they want to do."[36]

   Although it was crucial, supporters argued, to promote a specifically
American kind of fitness—one that was creative, engaging, and freely

sought by the nation's children—it was also of the utmost importance that such a program begin immediately and produce results. Children's physical fitness was an urgent matter because it was perceived as a national security issue. In the anxious political context, the public correlated the fitness of the country's children with the nation's survival in the Cold War. Citizens writing to the council warned that without improved fitness, the country would become the "next Red pole." As boxer Gene Tunney, who had participated in early PCYF planning meetings, put it, "Anything we can do to direct the activities and energies of young America, in a wholesome and healthful way, is a measure of national defense."[37]

Though concerned about what a national exercise program would entail, Americans were also intensely jealous of the Russians' medal achievements at the 1956 Olympics and of widely circulated news footage showing Russian youths exercising, thousands at a time.[38] Like many Americans of the era, physician and PCAC member Wilhelm Raab, who had visited the Soviet Union, was both afraid and envious of the next generation of Soviets. "Since my second trip . . . I am more than ever convinced of the frightening threat which the patiently and devotedly working, studying and self-sacrificing youth of the communist world poses to the future of our largely flabby, indifferent and cynical young people, the victims of an over-fed and, as it seems, over-ripe civilization."[39] For Raab and many others who saw fitness as a moral issue, well-trained bodies promised equally disciplined minds. By emphasizing children's mental development as well as their physical conditioning, the total fitness philosophy allowed MacCarthy and other officials to sidestep comparisons with Soviet and Nazi fitness programs while targeting character reform.

Perhaps the most telling example of the council's desire to match the Russians' perceived fitness levels was the creation of Youth Fitness Week. The PCYF created posters, sponsored commercials, and encouraged additional local programs for this week-long celebration of health, exercise, and sport. In the minds of council officials, media coverage of these American fitness activities could counteract Soviet May Day demonstrations, which were often reported on television. Youth Fitness Week, annually scheduled for the first week in May, functioned, as MacCarthy described it, as "a psychological weapon in the war of ideologies as the

Free World's voluntary celebration of 'May Day.'"[40] This direct challenge to Soviet fitness efforts illustrates how the framework of the fitness program had shifted from an antidelinquency measure to a national defense issue early in its existence. It also highlights the difficulty of MacCarthy's job: without the ability to enforce any kind of fitness mandate, he and his team had to find a way to make American children want to become fit of their own volition.

MacCarthy and his team were well aware of the irony that they were promoting fitness in order to compete with the Russians and maintain American superiority, all the while disavowing that they were like the Russians. To help American children become more fit, the PCYF would have to persuade youngsters and their parents to seek fitness, to engage in voluntary exercise, and to do it in a specifically American manner. While public fear that the PCYF would institute a mandatory physical fitness program gradually receded, council staff remained cognizant of the fact that if Americans were going to regain their physical superiority, it would have to be done through persuasion. Children and their parents would need to be convinced to participate in fitness because it was healthful and fun and because it was their civic duty. To make this happen, the PCYF would have to resort to the most American of methods: it would have to *sell* the idea of fitness to the public.

A second major challenge the PCYF faced was defining exactly what constituted *physical* fitness. Although the 1956 conference had established that fitness existed in many forms—physical fitness being only one aspect of the total concept—the council had very little information on which to base a definition of physical fitness and, by extension, total fitness. In the mid-1950s, there was little value in cultivating physical fitness for its own sake; for children, especially, fitness was the by-product of playing games with friends, participating in sports with teammates, or attending physical education classes at school. MacCarthy and those he collaborated with were guided by a general sense that physical activity was healthful, that it relieved stress (nervous tension, in the language of the day), and that team sports in particular were useful in the development of character. But the council lacked scientific information and feared both alienating potential allies and appearing to favor a particular group (such as an advocacy organization or manufacturer) over another. As a result, nearly any activity was considered fitness enhancing, from hunting to tennis to calisthenics to bowling.

As the PCYF's work was reported in the press, others wondered how fitness should be defined. *Sports Illustrated* summarized one of the major problems facing the new council:

> All the experts can say is that to be fit means to be able to carry on your daily life comfortably and have energy and strength left over for emergencies. This tells us little, because whose daily life are they talking about and what is the minimum fitness everyone should have? . . . For every test now in use there is at least one expert who disapproves of using it. To discover a scientific standard for fitness is one of the headaches the new fitness council and citizens' committee will face.[41]

The council's confusion over how to best promote physical fitness was not surprising. Research into the effects of physical activity on health was in its infancy.[42] As one physician put it, "Logic is on our side but statistical ammunition to prove the point is almost completely lacking."[43] PCAC member Dr. Donald Dukelow agreed, noting that "if pressed for an opinion [physicians] will say that some physical activity is desirable in normal well people. But they can rarely define what they mean by 'physical activity' or 'normal people.'"[44]

Given the difficulty of deciding what constituted fitness, it was not surprising that tests to gauge fitness were equally controversial. PCAC member Dr. William Walsh argued that "ample, available, applicable, accurate tests of physical fitness have not been determined."[45] The popular press similarly wondered about fitness testing and suggested that all the Kraus-Weber tests really measured was hamstring flexibility.[46] Widespread confusion about both the definition of fitness and how to measure it led the PCYF to try to be as inclusive as possible. MacCarthy and his team decided not to establish any formal definition of fitness; nor would the council support or endorse any definition created by another organization. In the absence of a scientific advisory council or the ability to fund research, this seems somewhat logical, but the decision to refuse to endorse fitness programs sponsored by other groups seems less so. Although physicians, physical educators, and recreation specialists took part in the council's activities, the PCYF refused to formally endorse any of the programs these qualified professionals were associated with. For example, Operation Fitness USA, an initiative of the American Association of Health, Physical Education and Recreation (AAHPER), eventually tested more than 20 million children in the United States and sixteen other countries, but it was never endorsed by the PCYF, despite having similar aims. AAHPER representatives participated in many council activities and linked patriotic ideas to fitness, as well as citing television and juvenile delinquency as reasons to support their cause, yet the PCYF declined to formally endorse the program because it recommended specific, absolute achievement goals for fitness. Given the council's refusal to support any particular type of activity or to make distinctions among team sports, calisthenics, and outdoor activities such as camping, shooting, and fishing, virtually any activity or community program could be considered a fitness activity. "In the eyes of the President's Council there are no minor sports," MacCarthy regularly told audiences.[47] Ultimately, such an inclusive stance weakened the council's ability to promote its message.

Nevertheless, the PCYF enjoyed widespread public support and was very successful in its efforts to increase awareness about the need for fitness. Americans were clamoring for information. Council publication runs were routinely exhausted, and television appearances by council staff were followed up by thousands of requests for additional information.[48] Everywhere, it seemed, parents were being encouraged to monitor and improve their children's fitness, but without more specific guidelines, this proved nearly impossible.

PCYF policies focused on developing awareness of the concept of personal fitness in general and encouraging parents and community leaders to initiate fitness programs (however they chose to define the term) in their towns. Typical of the activities the PCYF hoped to spur was the summer program organized by the city of Corpus Christi, Texas, in 1956. Sponsored by the recently created Corpus Christi Council for Physical Fitness and the local newspaper, the *Caller Times*, the program provided fitness training and testing to 600 children. Advertisements in the paper asked parents, "Can your boy chin himself? Chances are six to one that he can't!"[49] The town of Maywood, New Jersey, also organized a physical fitness committee. Mrs. M. Berger reported on the town's activities to PCYF officials: local committee members conducted physical fitness tests and found that 66 percent of the children tested were unfit, including Mrs. Berger's own son. The town addressed the problem by sponsoring fitness classes for children.[50] By 1960, thirty-seven states had held youth fitness conferences under the auspices of the governor's office, and nine others had held unofficial conferences.[51] During Youth Fitness Week in May, the PCYF stepped up its activities and publications. For Youth Fitness Week 1959, more than 175,000 Fitness Week kits were mailed to post offices, military installations, schools, and libraries.[52] Even the territories of Guam and Palau were included in the celebration of Youth Fitness Week.[53] As one PCAC member wrote of his state's efforts, "Nebraskans simply could not ignore the youth fitness movement as they were besieged on every side by television, radio and the newspapers."[54] The PCYF also worked with national nonprofit organizations such as 4-H, Jaycees, Junior Chamber of Commerce, Girl Scouts, Boy Scouts, and Camp Fire Girls, as well as the national governing offices of various religious denominations. Many of these groups adopted the theme of youth fitness for national meetings and covered fitness issues in local programs.[55]

Rarely, however, did the council's outreach efforts extend beyond the white middle class. The fitness levels of African American children received relatively little attention. African American congressman Adam Powell of New York visited the PCYF office in 1958 to discuss "youth fitness as it pertained to the negro population." MacCarthy reported that Powell "was satisfied that our planning and programming was conducted for all boys and girls."[56] The council's annual meeting sometimes included representatives from African American organizations, although the number varied over the years. In 1956, for example, officials from the National Association of Colored Women's Clubs and the National Congress of Colored Parents and Teachers attended, as did an African American sportswriter (out of a total of 149 participants).[57] In 1958, there were none. PCAC members attended annual meetings at their own expense, which could explain the varying level of participation. Sportswriter William D. Jackson of the *Cleveland Call and Post* wrote to Shane MacCarthy to explain that lack of funds prevented his newspaper from financing his trip to Washington for the 1960 meeting.[58]

Some black children may have been exposed to fitness awareness through their participation in African American branches of national youth organizations such as 4-H or Scouts, but there are no records indicating that the PCYF made any targeted efforts in the black community. Coverage of the PCYF fitness campaign in the black media was scant. The *Baltimore Afro-American* and the *Chicago Defender* mentioned youth fitness only rarely; *Jet* never mentioned it, nor did the *New Sign*, the newsletter of the Harlem YMCA, in spite of its own lineup of physical activities.

On the one hand, this neglect can be explained by the prevailing notion that the pursuit of fitness was viewed as an accommodation to a lifestyle of ease, something that most African Americans did not experience in the 1950s. The physical labor required of many in the working class, both black and white, was presumed to provide enough activity to ensure fitness. On the other hand, given the council's belief that fitness was the basis for a strong military, it seems foolish not to have included the African American community more fully in its awareness efforts. Black fighting units had been valuable assets during World War II and the Korean War. Council members may have presumed (recalling the notion of the "primitive other") that black bodies were already fit enough to fight. For their part, African Americans' participation in physical activities likely continued through this era, unaffected by the nationalistic lens of fitness.

In addition to nonprofit groups, the council cultivated relationships with corporations in an attempt to promote physical, though rarely total, fitness. The most successful of these partnerships was with General Mills, the manufacturer of Wheaties cereal. Wheaties had been associated with sports even before the fitness crisis, and General Mills was eager to be involved in the fitness campaign.[59] Harry Bullis, the CEO of General Mills, was a member of the PCAC, and Knox-Reeves, the Minneapolis advertising agency that directed the campaign, sent representatives to several PCYF meetings.[60] Wheaties' youth fitness campaign, led by former Olympic pole-vaulter and ordained minister Bob Richards, promoted athletics and fitness for children with the All-American Sports Fitness Tester, a fitness ability chart that appeared on the back of the cereal boxes in the late

1950s.[61] In the absence of widely available fitness standards, the testers were very popular with children.[62]

However, providing achievement charts and setting specific goals conflicted with the PCYF's all-inclusive fitness approach that accommodated all types of activities and all levels of achievement. After spending a good deal of time working with General Mills to promote fitness, the PCYF was annoyed that the testers used absolute criteria to gauge fitness, but it decided that issuing a corrective press release would be pointless.[63] The council was forced to accept the fact that working with outside sponsors meant that these groups would adapt the fitness message to their own needs, and in many cases, that meant promoting physical fitness over total fitness.

From the start, PCYF planners imagined children in terms of market. Early in the planning process, Bob King, assistant to President Eisenhower, advised Vice President Nixon that the council's work should be confined to "sales promotion."[64] MacCarthy was thinking along these same lines and asked a subordinate to order a copy of marketing guru Eugene Gilbert's influential book *Advertising and Marketing to Young People*.[65] By midcentury, adolescent baby boomers were well on their way to constituting a distinct market demographic.[66] Sales of child-related products such as diapers, toys, and sporting goods rose dramatically between the late 1940s and late 1950s.[67] The PCYF recognized this trend. The fitness campaign and the products associated with it would be just another Madison Avenue commodity taking advantage of the youth-oriented decade.

The council actively worked to get businesses interested in using fitness as a platform to sell their goods and held workshops for interested companies. In addition to increased sales, manufacturers would benefit by associating their work with patriotic causes and creating corporate goodwill. The PCYF cooperated with reporter Victor Gold, who wrote an article for the trade publication the *Public Relations Journal* that outlined the public-private partnerships the council had embarked on and provided a list of the types of products PCYF officials would be most interested in associating with the fitness message: personal items such as soap, toothpaste, and apparel; those with a sports or outdoors connotation; and "special promotions aimed at the expanding young adult market."[68] Council

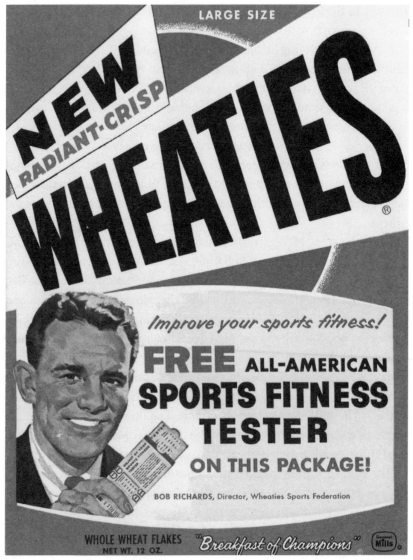

General Mills printed a fitness tester on boxes of Wheaties cereal in 1959 to encourage children to become physically fit. Although General Mills was an active participant in the PCYF's national campaign, like all the council's corporate partners, it chose to promote physical rather than "total" fitness. (Courtesy of General Mills Archives)

General Mills fitness tester. (Courtesy of General Mills Archives)

staff organized a number of workshops with leaders of the business community to brainstorm about ways to incorporate the fitness message into advertising and other media. In 1960, the PCYF hosted a forum where public relations professional Robert M. Hoffman gave a talk entitled "Telling and Selling the Fitness Story." In his lengthy presentation, Hoffman lectured the assembled group on the creation of preference through careful marketing. Already imagining fitness as a commodity, he encouraged listeners to market fitness like any other product: "We must now make our prospects pant to buy our product. We must convince them that it is the

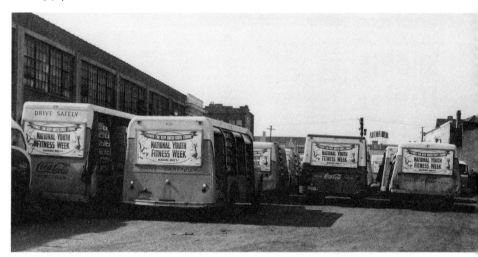

In honor of Youth Fitness Week 1960, one Cleveland Coca-Cola distributor decorated his entire fleet of delivery vehicles to promote fitness. Independent, voluntary displays of support such as this one attest to the warm public response to the fitness message. (Records of the President's Council on Physical Fitness, National Archives)

most desirable thing in the world, that they can't live without it, that it is the most important purchase of their entire lives. . . . We must make them want fitness the way every teenager yearns for a blue convertible."[69]

Corporate involvement in fitness promotion took on a variety of guises. During Youth Fitness Week 1960, one Cleveland Coca-Cola distributor covered his entire distribution fleet in promotional advertising that proclaimed, "Fitness Can Keep United States Strong."[70] In the Washington, D.C., area, Safeway grocery stores ran a newspaper advertisement proclaiming, "Youth fitness means a sound mind in a sound body, eat well to keep well, shop Safeway."[71] In some cases, fitness promotion came about thanks to the involvement of well-connected PCAC members. Carter Burgess, advisory committee chair and CEO of Trans World Airlines, used the TWA marquee on Broadway to promote fitness.[72] A year later, as the newly installed CEO of American Machine and Foundry, owner of the largest chain of bowling alleys in the nation, Burgess allowed the company's regular advertising minutes to be filled with fitness spots during Youth Fitness Week and distributed posters featuring comic strip character Joe Palooka bowling "for fitness, for health, for family fun."[73] Perhaps the most unusual promotion technique was embarked on by Baume Ben-Gué (now known as BenGay ointment). Between 1958 and 1960, the brand owners, in collaboration with advertising agency William Esty Inc., sponsored an attractive young masseuse, Dixie Qualset, to make public appearances as Miss Youth Fitness. In that capacity, she toured a number of cities offering massages, engaging the public in conversations about fitness, and attending sporting events, women's club lunches, and chamber of commerce meetings, as well as stopping at radio stations and newspapers along the way.[74] In New York, for example, she lunched with spouses of the city's professional athletes.[75] In Milwaukee, she made an appearance at a wrestling match.[76] Chosen for her petite stature and physical appeal, Qualset had "a magnificently developed set of pectoral muscles," as a reporter for the *New York Times* wryly observed.[77] Qualset also appeared as Miss Youth Fitness on the television quiz shows *To Tell the Truth* and *What's My Line?*[78] Although Qualset had been briefed at PCYF offices before embarking on her tour, the relationship, like others the council maintained with corporate promoters, was delicate. While acknowledging that her work was beneficial, the council also distanced itself from her efforts. Wrote one staffer, the tour "is done with our knowledge and policy orientation, but is neither endorsed nor sponsored by the Council."[79]

The relationships the council entertained with corporate sponsors expanded the scope of the fitness campaign beyond simple public information, but the promotion of physical fitness overshadowed the council's total fitness message. Viewed from a wider perspective, however, this additional publicity extended the reach of the physical fitness message, setting a foundation of awareness in a whole generation of baby boomers and their parents. While fitness messages were focused on children, awareness messages were directed primarily at adults, who followed fitness discussions in the media. Because of the council's work, two generations of Americans became familiar with the notion that the body required maintenance in the form of physical activity, and it was this growing conviction that helped propel the development of a new fitness industry in the following decade.

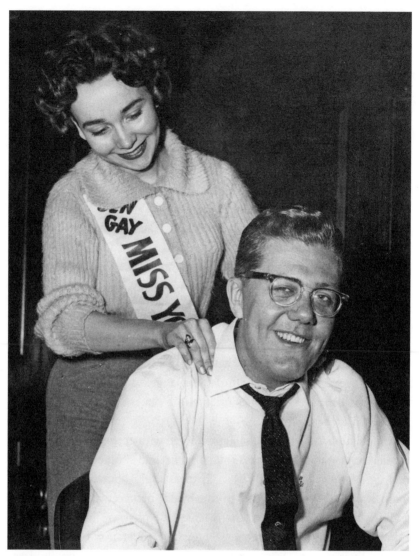

Masseuse Dixie Qualset with journalist Jack Lavin at the Palmer House in Chicago in 1959. The maker of BenGay ointment sponsored a national publicity tour for Qualset, who traveled around the country promoting physical fitness. She made stops at charity and sports events and appeared on What's My Line? and To Tell the Truth as Miss Youth Fitness. (Collection of the author)

MOTHERS AND FATHERS OF TOMORROW

In addition to promoting character reform to curb juvenile delinquency and physical fitness to form fit bodies, the total fitness philosophy—with its emphasis on social and emotional fitness—worked to reinforce a heterosexual family structure and traditional gender roles. As one PCAC member explained, "[It's] true, we approve [of] and encourage athletics, but our real objective is a program that helps youth to become fit as scientists, professional people, soldiers, workers, farmers, business managers, merchants, financiers—and above all, as husbands and wives, mothers and fathers of tomorrow."[80]

Encouraging proper gender role development was particularly important in postwar America, given the changes that ensued when extended urban families transitioned to nuclear suburban families. As women returned to the home following wartime employment and men returned to the traditional role of breadwinner, children were left alone with their mothers in this new suburban context. Experts fretted that sons would receive too little paternal attention and too much maternal affection. Fear of "momism," a term coined by Philip Wylie in his best seller *Generation of Vipers*, was reflected in PCYF literature and correspondence.

As a traditionally male domain, fitness in the form of sports programs was viewed as a welcome antidote to mothers' influence. As one municipal recreation supervisor put it, "We must go back to the home and get Dad interested in his boy, at the school, on the playground and on the ball field. . . . Send out a challenge to Dads all over the country. It is their job!"[81] Similarly, *New York Times Magazine* writer Dorothy Barclay feared that mothers would have a disproportionate influence over their sons' recreation at home: "The overanxious mother hampers her offspring by worried warnings and limitations of his movements. Because she is fearful for his safety she closely controls his activities. As a result, such a child may become timid, muscularly weak and tense."[82] Even the American Medical Association took up the issue, warning that parental overprotection in general could be more psychically dangerous than any physical injury, stating in a JAMA editorial that "medicine recognizes that a fractured ankle may leave less of a scar than a personality frustrated by reason of parental timidity in contact sports."[83]

Although PCYF literature paid equal attention to boys and girls, it was clear that fitness served two different, gender-specific goals. Boys, who would become the next generation of soldiers, required fitness to protect the nation in future military conflicts and then to become fathers, in both biological and emotional terms. For boys, total fitness efforts were directed toward creating strength, hardiness, mental fortitude, and manliness. The council's goals for girls were more narrow, focusing primarily on the cultivation of health for reproductive purposes—in other words, on their ability to become "Republican mothers," or women whose importance derived from their ability to produce and then properly rear sons for the benefit of the nation.[84] As MacCarthy told one audience, "Our goal . . . looks toward healthful, vital, masculine men and active, healthful, vital, feminine women who can mother a vigorous generation."[85] Elaine Tyler May has established that reproduction was a patriotic act during the Cold War; childbearing and attentive parenting were considered important aspects of good citizenship.[86] Procreation demonstrated one's investment in the nation, on both a personal and a public scale. In its focus on creating healthy bodies for reproduction, the total fitness philosophy united the intimate with the civic. The poster distributed to promote National Fitness Week in 1960 made it clear that youngsters' bodies were just as important for the role they played in the home as in the defense of the nation. Bearing the slogan "Fitness Can Keep US Strong"—with "US" meaning both "United States" and "us"—and depicting the silhouette of a boy and a girl holding hands superimposed on the silhouette of a man and a woman holding hands, the poster linked fitness with heterosexuality and hinted at the production of generations to come.[87]

A second aspect of the emotional fitness the PCYF tried to promote was based on its collective opinion that life in mid-twentieth-century America was fundamentally more stressful than in the past. Council officials believed that one result of the new environment was an increase in mental illness among young people.[88] Physical activity was imagined to be a therapeutic technique that could help soothe "the inevitable by-product of our present tense and mechanical method of living."[89] In the absence of yesteryear's physical outlets for stress, new skills were necessary to adapt to the new era. Throughout its correspondence and publications, the coun-

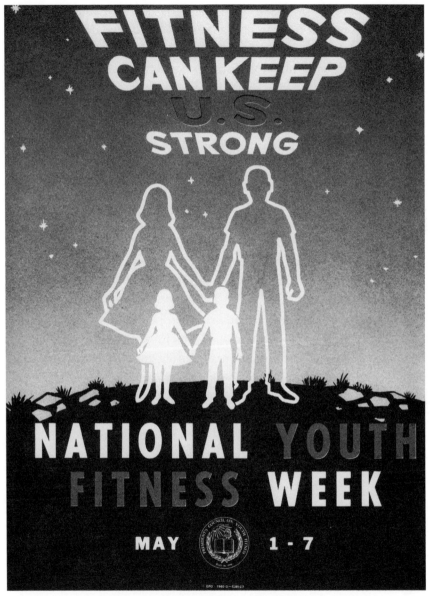

The council's total fitness message, with its emphasis on good conduct, the responsibilities of citizenship, and healthy bodies, is evident in this 1960 poster for Youth Fitness Week. PCYF organizers viewed fitness as a quality necessary for the reproduction of future generations. (Records of the President's Council on Physical Fitness, National Archives)

cil emphasized the benefits of physical fitness, arguing that exercise and sports "will remain through life as 'safety valves' for relieving the pressures of high tension living."[90]

The promotion of physical activity as a coping mechanism also supported the council's interest in healthy gender role development and procreation. At midcentury, homosexuality was imagined to be a condition that could develop under the right circumstances, especially when an individual suffered from too much emotional stress. According to sociologist Lester Kirkendall, a well-known sex education expert of the period, homosexuals were "blocked in their normal development by conflicts. . . . A combination of factors thus produces the homosexual, an individual who might with better fortune have followed the normal processes of maturing and growing up."[91] Given the belief that "normal" sexual development was dependent on good mental health and that physical activity played a role in its achievement, total fitness also functioned as a means to curb homosexuality.

Although messages about emotional and social fitness played relatively minor roles in the PCYF's promotion of total fitness, they demonstrate its interest in youth reform on a grand scale and illustrate that no area of youth experience was beyond its purview. MacCarthy and his team envisioned physical fitness, and the social and emotional benefits associated with it, as a habit that would help young people reach adulthood with the ability to adjust to their rapidly changing world and ensure the proper development of a new generation of marriage partners, parents, and citizens.

"A NEW SOFTNESS"

In the first five years following World War II, spending on household appliances and furnishings grew 240 percent, flooding American homes with a variety of devices designed to make life more comfortable.[92] By 1960, 87 percent of American homes had televisions, 75 percent of American families owned cars, and 75 percent owned washing machines.[93] The new crop of household appliances that Americans had labeled "push-button gadgets" represented a successful economy and, during the Cold War, the triumph of democracy over communism. Just how strongly Americans identified material goods as symbols of progress and freedom was made clear during Vice President Nixon's trip to Moscow in 1959. There, Nixon engaged Nikita Khrushchev in what became known as the "kitchen debate." As they toured a model home at the American National Exhibition, Nixon told a disbelieving Khrushchev of a society where even "average workers" could easily afford consumer goods such as homes, automobiles, and televisions. For the vice president, the supremacy of the American political system over the Soviet one was proved not by free elections, the space race, or military strength but by how consumers lived.[94]

One reason the Kraus-Hirschland report was so troubling, then, was the fact that the same goods Americans used to justify the rightness of democracy and the free market were being indicted as the cause of their physical unfitness. Kraus and Hirschland had blamed American children's poor fitness on the fruits of the U.S. economic system. The report issued after the 1956 meeting in Annapolis also blamed modern life, noting, "Our scientific and technological advances of today, while bringing an ease to living, deprive us of needed physical activity."[95] Newspapers and magazines similarly weighed in on how lifestyles had changed over the decades. Central heating had rendered wood chopping unnecessary, cars and school buses reduced walking dramatically, television meant that leisure time was spent indoors, and conveniences such as electric washers, dishwashers, can openers, and vacuum cleaners reduced household labor.[96] While such luxuries represented prosperity, they were also dangerous in that they could make citizens lazy and physically unfit. Rugged American bodies of the past had not been shaped by ease and convenience.

Though the PCYF insisted that it was not against progress or modern-day conveniences, much of its rhetoric cast economic prosperity and increased leisure time in terms of sin, sloth, and gluttony and warned that without intervention, the nation would be in jeopardy. MacCarthy and his correspondents frequently made comparisons between the Roman Empire and the United States. As one senator explained to his constituents, "If we are going to retain our world leadership, we cannot permit this condition [unfitness] to continue. Mighty Rome collapsed when it lost its physical health. A flabby nation physically becomes a flabby nation mentally and spiritually."[97] Although material abundance functioned as evidence of American superiority, it was clear that prosperity could also endanger the country's continued survival. As PCYF organizers saw the situation, it was not their job to advocate a return to a frontier existence or to convince Americans to consume less; they could only encourage a lifestyle that accommodated both the fruits of the nation's economy and new fitness habits to guarantee the physical and mental edge previously achieved through life in a rough-and-tumble environment.

Fitness advocates were quick to condemn anything that reduced physical activity, but no object received as much scorn as the television, which not only invited sedentary behavior but also, they believed, dulled the mind. In the decade between 1950 and 1960, the number of American households with television sets jumped from 1 million to 50 million.[98] Television was viewed as particularly dangerous because it encouraged youngsters to spend their leisure time inside rather than engaging in outdoor play or sports. For the PCYF, the televising of sporting events was doubly troubling because children could choose to stay home and watch rather than participating themselves. Just as fitness activities were imagined to bestow health, television was seen as having the potential to make children ill. Historian Tom Englehardt has cataloged a number of childhood illnesses that were thought to result from too much television time: "TV squint," which caused eyestrain; "TV bottom," a result of physical inactivity; "frogitis," inner thigh strain as a result of sitting in a W position; "TV tummy," an upset stomach resulting from too much excitement; "TV jaw," developed when the hands propped up the head; and "tired child syndrome," with symptoms including chronic fatigue, headaches, and vomiting.[99] Similarly, Lynn Spigel's research on early television documented "telebugeye," a disorder that rendered children "pale, weak and stupid-looking."[100] PCYF officials shared the belief that television contributed to poor health, although their preferred term was "spectatoritis," which included the cinema as well.

It was not just the inactivity of television watching that bothered the council and its supporters; they were also disturbed by the passive nature of viewing. *Cosmopolitan* charged that "today's children flick a switch and expect to be entertained. They do nothing but absorb."[101] PCYF staff members believed that television robbed children of their capacity for active play and creative thinking. They and other critics feared that "the one-eyed hypnotic monster" somehow had the power to control children's

minds.[102] Certain individuals, it was imagined, might be overly susceptible to television programming, possibly reenacting the violence they
saw on the screen.[103] Undoubtedly, council members envisioned parallels
between passivity and communism. Whereas a democratic government
required the participation of active, thinking citizens (as Americans imagined themselves to be), communism encouraged passive, submissive subjects (like the Russians). The deleterious effects of television and soft living in general, and their combined influence on the American nation, were
topics that gave shape to fitness discussions and provided a framework
for understanding why the Kraus-Hirschland report sparked such heated
controversy. The nation's unfitness problem, particularly as it pertained to
civilians, was troubling because the impact on the next generation could
not be predicted. Would Americans of the future be less capable of independent thinking and therefore more susceptible to communist ideology?
Would they be able to fulfill their duties as voters and members of the community? How would their bodies function as new material conveniences
continued to arrive on the market? When it came to the military, however,
these theoretical questions gave way to the belief that the effects of unfitness were already being felt in very dangerous ways.

Pampered Soldiers

Popular media discussions of the Kraus-Weber tests almost always mentioned the military in connection with children's fitness.[104] The Kraus-
Hirschland report seemed to shed light on the causes of both recent and
long-term problems plaguing the nation's armed forces. Many Americans
believed that the country's soldiers were weaker than at any point in history, and the media frequently reminded readers that in each successive
military intervention beginning with World War I, increasing numbers of
American men had been found unfit for military duty.

Reports during World War I estimated that 37 percent of inductees had
been rejected for physical defects, leading the *Saturday Evening Post* to la-
ment that the war had "dispelled several of our national illusions . . . with
its enlistments and its draft, gradually it began to drift in on us that we were
going to have trouble in getting an army."[105] During World War II, the government released rejection figures at regular intervals. Between 1940 and

1945, the percentage of men rejected for service ranged from 35 percent to 50 percent, leading President Roosevelt to express public concern about the number of rejections and the nation's health in general. Ultimately, 6.5 million American men were rejected for service.[106] During the Korean War, out of the 4 million young men examined for draft registration between 1948 and 1955, slightly more than 2 million were rejected on physical and mental grounds—52 percent. Even though these figures were somewhat misleading, in that they did not include the large number of men who volunteered for service, they gained widespread currency.[107] Moreover, these figures were perceived as particularly problematic, given the number of men available for duty in the far more populous Soviet Union and China.[108]

The Korean War rejection rates were viewed as part of a pattern of increasing national softness exacerbated by postwar affluence. The cause of the problem, according to one general, was not that American men had been "neglected" but that they had been "pampered."[109] Though serious, the physical problems associated with soldiers' lack of fitness had known solutions: boot camp, drills, and calisthenics could reform soft bodies. Far more complicated was the issue of the mental, moral, and character problems present in the new generation. As the *Saturday Evening Post* observed in an article about the nation's soldiers, the high standard of living and economic security of the previous half century had "robbed too many of some of the native American birthrights—daring, incentive, initiative, push, aggressiveness, self-dependence. We have changed from a 'have-not' to a 'have' nation—but we are vulnerable like all the rich and surfeited empires and kingdoms of the past to the slow corrosion of luxury, the attrition of ease."[110] Anecdotal claims like these, which clearly focused on nonphysical changes, were backed up by more specific evidence that the military was experiencing conduct and behavioral problems. A large number of courts-martial, a significant number of deserters, and a growing military prison population were cited as evidence of a decline in military standards.[111] Above all, the perception of a troubled military was influenced by the conduct of prisoners of war during and in the aftermath of the Korean War, which had ended in 1953.

During the Korean War, 7,190 Americans were taken prisoner and sent to twenty prison camps; of these, 2,730 men died in the camps.[112] The fact that 38 percent of American POWs died—a rate higher than in any other war in U.S. history—was interpreted not as a commentary on harsh camp conditions but rather as a failure on the part of the soldiers and their training.[113] Of the soldiers who survived, many had reportedly collaborated with the enemy; a military investigation into POW conduct found that one-third of the 4,428 men held captive had capitulated to enemy demands in some way. The offenses ranged from "writing anti-American propaganda and informing on comrades" to "broadcasting Christmas greetings home" and stating that they were being well treated.[114] Even among those soldiers not found guilty of collaborating, reports of disrespect for superiors, lack of unit cohesiveness, failure to maintain the chain of command, and even failure to attempt to escape were cited as evidence that something had gone awry in their military training to allow such behavior.[115] The highly publicized trial of Sergeant James C. Gallagher, who was accused of collaborating with the enemy and murdering three American soldiers in a Korean POW camp, added to the flood of poor press for returning American soldiers.[116]

Journalist Eugene Kinkead wrote a lengthy article for the *New Yorker* (as well as a subsequent book) detailing the military's investigation into POW conduct and explaining how Chinese and Korean captors convinced American soldiers to break ranks, hoard food, and "convert" to communism. Kinkead interviewed Major Clarence L. Anderson, a former POW and American military physician, who blamed an "almost universal inability of the prisoners to adjust to a primitive situation. 'They lacked the old Yankee resourcefulness,'" he said. "'This was partly—but only partly, I believe—the result of the psychic shock of being captured. It was also, I think, the result of some new failure in the childhood and adolescent training of our young men—a new softness.'"[117] Kinkead's report described men who seemed to believe that they were no longer part of a military unit once they were captured, men who no longer had a sense of self-sufficiency and who had reverted to a state of near helplessness that Anderson termed "give-up-itis." Anderson also noticed that older POWs (meaning those who had not enjoyed lives of abundance) fared better than younger ones in the camps, and he regretted that the American soldiers had been treated so well during training.[118] Kinkead emphasized that the problems in Korea had been preventable, noting that military forces from other nations had fared better than American soldiers; he concluded that a lack of discipline and hardiness was to blame. The PCYF embraced this opinion, inviting Kinkead to speak at a forum for communications professionals in 1960.[119]

Of all the conduct-related issues military officials faced, none was more chilling than the decision of twenty-one American POWs to remain behind the Iron Curtain rather than return home. Final peace negotiations had hinged on whether prisoners on both sides would be compelled to return to their country of origin or could choose another destination. In holding out for the latter, American officials had hoped to secure a moral victory by allowing the approximately 50,000 North Korean and Chinese prisoners the opportunity to remain in South Korea, never suspecting that some of their own compatriots might choose not to return to the United States. When twenty-three did so (two men ultimately decided to accept repatriation), the American public surmised that the only possible explanation was brainwashing.[120]

Introduced in 1951 by journalist and probable CIA operative Edward Hunter, the term *brainwashing* had gained quick political and popular currency. As one writer put it, the concept "burst like a bombshell upon the American consciousness during the Korean War."[121] Accounts from returning POWs detailed political indoctrination and forced confessions that were obtained through what *Time* called "Communist mental torture." Colonel Frank Schwable, a pilot shot down over Korea, had made a false confession that Americans were using germ warfare; he described being subjected to solitary confinement, sleep deprivation, temperature extremes, and living "like an animal wallowing around in dirt and filth."[122] Other soldiers had been coerced into broadcasting false confessions and expressing sympathy with communist ideology.[123] Stories also circulated that American soldiers had been captured, indoctrinated, and then returned to the front lines, where they worked to convince others to desert.[124]

For nearly the entire decade, and peaking during the formative years of the PCYF, brainwashing and mind control were popularized in legal proceedings and governmental investigations, nonfiction books about the twenty-one "turncoats," and memoirs written by former captives.[125] These topics also became a central part of popular culture, forming the backdrop for fictional books, television specials, and Hollywood films, including the best known of the genre, *The Manchurian Candidate*, a 1962 movie based on the 1958 novel.[126] The public conversation about brainwashing reflected the belief that the nature of war had changed. The Korean War had ushered in an era of total warfare that was fought not only on the battlefields but also in the minds of men. The war's unsatisfying conclusion, POWs' comportment, and widespread doubt about the military's ability to achieve victory led to a period of American soul-searching. Historian Susan Carruthers has argued that the weakness of soldiers abroad was viewed as evidence of weakness at home, pointing out that POW behavior functioned as a "referendum on national character" that "prompted a vote of no confidence in the entire postwar generation."[127]

Youth fitness policy, then, was a terrain where anxieties related to material abundance, gender roles, physical fitness, and mental preparedness for combat played out. Seen in this context, the PCYF's emphasis on total fitness, rather than physical fitness, is understandable. In a speech in New Jersey, MacCarthy specifically linked poor military conduct in Korea to the need for total fitness. Repeating the charges leveled by Kinkead and other critics, such as the prisoners' failure to escape and their submission "to the wiles of the Communist enemy," MacCarthy blamed "ease, luxury and human inactivity" for a "lack of leadership, courage and discipline" among Korean War soldiers. In addition, MacCarthy asserted that four out of ten young people dropped out of college because of a "lack of willpower" and stated that 60 percent of the nation's hospital beds were filled with patients who suffered from mental health problems. MacCarthy's remarks placed character development and mental health under the same umbrella, illustrating the type of thinking that led the PCYF to imagine that its total fitness policy might remedy all that ailed postwar America.[128]

By far, the strongest evidence that events in Korea played a role in the PCYF's total fitness initiative was the appointment of Carter Burgess as head of the PCAC. As assistant secretary of defense for manpower and personnel from 1955 to 1957, Burgess had worked closely on matters relating to the POWs held in Korea. In fact, Burgess had chaired the committee investigating POW conduct and had led the production of its report on American POWs throughout history.[129] The committee's most significant accomplishment was the creation of the military code of conduct in July 1955, which clarified the obligations of service members being held by an enemy.[130] The six-part oath—best known for its provision that service members disclose only "name, rank, service number and date of birth" if captured—was written as a pledge of sorts that directly addressed the charges of poor behavior in Korea. The code emphasized soldiers' responsibility to resist the enemy, their duty to attempt to escape, not accept special treatment, and "keep faith with . . . fellow prisoners." It also indirectly addressed mind control: "I will never surrender my own free will. If in command I will never surrender my men while they have the means to resist."[131]

The code was designed to solve the conduct problem the committee had been assigned to study. Its final report described a new kind of "all inclusive" warfare that blurred the boundary between civilian and military life. "Today there are no distant front lines, remote no man's lands, far-off rear areas. The home front is but an extension of the fighting front."[132] The committee espoused a view that modern warfare could be fought successfully only by soldiers who had started preparing early in civilian life—even during childhood. The report recommended the development of "spiritual and educational bulwarks against enemy political indoctrination" and suggested a partnership with the Department of Health, Education, and Welfare for "pre-service training." In short, the POW committee concluded that training for military service needed to begin long before boot camp.[133]

Although Burgess stepped down from his Defense Department post prior to beginning his work with the PCAC, his opinions on the need to prepare for total warfare did not change during his tenure as advisory committee chair. He reminded the audience assembled at the 1957 PCYF conference at West Point of the recently established military code of conduct and emphasized that the physical and mental attributes required by soldiers in the line of duty were "not something that can be acquired overnight—nor even after one enters into the ranks for his country's freedom." "Fitness," he informed the audience, "begins in the high chair!"[134] Burgess asked how a nation could demand fitness during war when peacetime fitness programs were nonexistent. This logical question helps explain the connection between events in Korea and PCYF programming. In the minds of organizers, it simply was not possible to achieve military preparedness for Cold War threats with only short-term measures such as boot camp. The council's attempt to promote total fitness failed miserably, however.

PROMOTING TOTAL FITNESS

If promoting physical fitness proved difficult, defining and promoting total fitness turned out to be a herculean task. Though the PCYF was never able to come to an agreement on a definition of physical fitness or a way to measure it, the council was nevertheless able to promote it well because physical fitness was, generally speaking, a concept with which the public had some familiarity. The PCYF managed to convince corporations, associations, and parents that it was important to promote fitness, and it had to acquiesce when these activities tended to focus on the physical. Promoting total fitness was another matter entirely. Attempts to promote mental, moral, social, and other nonphysical types of fitness were clumsy and ill conceived. Other than raising vague notions of ethics, morals, good character, and self-discipline in promotional literature, PCYF officials did little to define these other kinds of fitness or explain how to achieve them. PCYF officials could not even succinctly define total fitness for themselves. MacCarthy entered into negotiations with the Ad Council to develop a national advertising campaign, but plans fell through when it became clear that the PCYF could not clearly articulate a total fitness philosophy.[135] Among council staff and committee members and in PCYF publications, ideas of total fitness were most often expressed in the context of larger discussions about the moral and ethical qualities that physical fitness could encourage. One of the few council publications that addressed total fitness was more notable for its lengthy description of "unfit" qualities than its promotion of total fitness: "Can we call fit . . . the boy who cheats in school or on the basketball court? The girl whose will is such that she is afraid to learn to swim, or to dance? . . . The boy who will only participate when he is the captain, or the chief?"[136] The total fitness philosophy seemed to echo general principles of sportsmanship, but how these ideals could be taught was left to the reader's imagination.

The total fitness philosophy was visible more specifically in the council's work with organized religion. The PCYF reached out to the national offices of various religious denominations to encourage total fitness programs in churches and synagogues. These efforts entailed suggesting sermons for Youth Fitness Week, circulating a special youth fitness prayer, and distributing posters for church bulletin boards. In addition, the PCYF sponsored a workshop for leaders of religious organizations to explore how total fitness could be incorporated into their youth programs.[137] Council publications outlined the reasons why religion was important to the total fitness mission rather than how to develop fitness.[138] As with physical fitness, the council preferred to leave the specifics to others. Catholics and Mormons were particularly active in PCYF meetings at the national level. The Church of Latter-Day Saints, with its already extensive youth programming, was especially receptive to total fitness ideas. During Youth Fitness Week 1959, more than 1 million Mormons received "direct instruction from the Church to emphasize and employ the materials we are providing for them during Youth Fitness Week."[139] In addition, Mormon youth received special fitness messages delivered via "wire hook-up" over a fourteen-week period in early 1960.[140]

Another way the PCYF tried to promote total fitness was to downplay physical fitness as the most desirable type of fitness, creating documents and advertising that referred simply to "fitness." Drafts of radio spots that ran during Youth Fitness Week 1958 reveal that the PCYF removed terms such as "physical" and "bodies" so that, in some cases, there was no mention of physical exercise at all.[141] Shane MacCarthy explained this effort as an attempt to promote total fitness: "I am sure you have noticed how careful we are in our publications about not placing the word 'physical' in front of 'fitness.' For us, fitness contains mental, emotional, social and spiritual as well as physical components."[142] More blatant attempts to de-emphasize physical fitness sometimes seemed to criticize those who had heeded the council's message about physical development. A poster designed for widespread distribution obliquely hinted at the council's heterosexual aims, stating, "The President's Council is not trying to develop a race of piano lifters or jungle fighters, nor of muscle molls or amazons."[143] But simply promoting "fitness" as opposed to "physical fitness" and criticizing a preoccupation with one's body did not transmit the total fitness message. Without programming to explain how to achieve other facets of fitness, the public seized on the PCYF's most accessible message: the promotion of physical fitness.

Some PCAC members were dismayed by this failure to promote total fitness. After reading the PCYF's report on the annual meeting at West Point, one disconcerted physician was surprised at how little attention total fitness had received. "The general tone of the paper is one of physical strength and fitness with only lip service and bare mention of the really more important emotional and spiritual fitness," he wrote in a letter.[144] Three years into the fitness campaign, it was evident that the PCYF had failed to adequately address total fitness and that physical fitness issues were overshadowing moral, social, and other concerns. At least one advisory committee member resigned in frustration at the lack of total fitness programming. Philip Broughton, secretary of the Mellon Trust, sent Mac-Carthy a letter that complained, "I also have somewhat the feeling that I am out of step with the rest of the brigade. . . . All the material that comes into my office from various organizations . . . is related to the calisthenics, sports, muscle building aspects of 'fitness.' . . . Sometimes I get the impression that these outright physical education boys so overwhelm the President's Citizens Advisory Committee that I am pretty irrelevant."[145]

Without a precise definition and a strategic plan to implement total fitness, the PCYF could never realize its vision of youth reform and military preparedness. The council's inability to distinguish total fitness from physical fitness resulted in a public information campaign that was vague and ill defined from the start. MacCarthy and his team were immensely successful in one aspect of total fitness, however: increasing the public's awareness of physical fitness.

MacCarthy ended his term as executive director of the PCYF in 1961. The nation had elected a new president, and it was clear that fitness promotion efforts by the federal government were about to change course. Even before taking office, John F. Kennedy addressed the fitness problem in a *Sports Illustrated* article that criticized the lack of improvement in the physical fitness of American children over the past five years.[146] Though his words about fitness, national security, and the role of citizen-soldiers in a democracy were remarkably similar to PCYF rhetoric, Kennedy made it clear that his administration's fitness efforts would focus on the physical.

After his inauguration, he implemented this policy by changing the name of the organization to the President's Council on *Physical* Fitness and appointing University of Oklahoma football coach Charles "Bud" Wilkinson as director. Total fitness was cast aside in favor of vim, "vigah," competitive sports, and achievement tests.

Kennedy infused both personal interest and more powerful programming into fitness efforts during his short administration. The personalized nature of his appeals for fitness on television and radio made an impact on the public that MacCarthy's team had failed to achieve: despite multiple requests by the PCYF, Eisenhower had never addressed the nation about fitness.[147] Nor had the PCYF ever been well funded. From the start, Eisenhower had imagined that governmental efforts to promote fitness would come from private volunteer sources.[148] During his administration, no direct funds were ever secured to ensure the continued existence of the PCYF or its programs. Two bills were introduced in Congress in 1958 that requested funds for fitness endeavors, but both died in committee.[149] Funding to run the PCYF office was dependent on the largesse of sponsoring cabinet departments and the executive branch.[150] For these reasons, and despite the tireless efforts of Shane MacCarthy and his energetic staff, the President's Council on Youth Fitness, the first extensive governmental effort to promote fitness for civilians, was overshadowed by the physical fitness efforts of the next administration. But the success of these later efforts was due in large part to the foundation of awareness laid by the MacCarthy team.

Despite numerous obstacles, the PCYF succeeded in its goal of increasing awareness of physical fitness in the United States. By the late 1950s, Americans were familiar with the notion of personal physical fitness and had begun to integrate exercise into their lives—or at least they had started to think about how they might do this. In the decades to come, governmental efforts to promote fitness, especially those that focused on duty to the detriment of fun, would become less important as for-profit exercise entrepreneurs, sporting goods manufacturers, and consumer health authorities grew in number and importance—due, at least in part, to the constant promotional efforts of the PCYF. As one Texas sporting goods merchant reported in 1959, the fitness campaign had increased both sales and interest: "We feel the need for personal fitness is really beginning to be recognized. We have noticed considerable interest locally in health studios, gymnasium equipment and home exerciser sets. Our own sales of sweat clothing doubled in recent months as a result of a public awakening to more exercising."[151] Fitness impresario Vic Tanny, who owned a chain of gyms, also noticed a connection between the council's efforts and the burgeoning commercial fitness industry, observing, "The Russians? Nuts! All that our people need is regular workouts at my gyms and they can lick everyone's father."[152]

For Shane MacCarthy and supporters of the PCYF, discussions of physical activity had provided a forum for the critique of consumption. The fitness of bodies functioned as an index to the nation's well-being, even before the health benefits of physical activity were fully known. The midcentury period marked the start of a new era in which the body's able functioning could no longer be taken for granted. Accepting the conveniences of modern living meant that maintaining physical well-being would require conscious thought and attention. Consumers wouldn't have to look far for solutions, however. In subsequent years, thanks to the efforts of the PCYF, the same consumer culture that had created the problem of soft living would provide answers in the form of health clubs and exercise shows, records, and machines.

"YOUR HONEYMOON FIGURE"

WOMEN'S WEIGHT REDUCTION AND EXERCISE IN THE 1960S

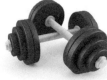

2

If fear of "softness" provided the context for Americans'
interest in exercise in the 1950s, in the following decade it
was concern about obesity that created a favorable climate
for the continuing expansion of fitness culture. Gradually,
the patriotic fervor surrounding youth fitness yielded to
a new era in which everyone's bodies came under intense
scrutiny—especially those of women. Peter Wyden, executive editor at *Ladies' Home Journal*, surveyed the new culture
of "Dietland, U.S.A." in a 1965 book he called *The Overweight
Society*. In sixteen chapters that bear an amazing resem-
blance to the culture of weight loss in twenty-first-century
America, Wyden explored the new terrain of appetite suppressants and liquid meal replacement drinks, spas and
exercise trends, the food industry's need to increase consumption for profit, and conflicting nutritional theories.
Although Wyden's book employed a tongue-in-cheek tone,
it took its subject quite seriously. Thinness, Wyden wrote, is
"an important ambition because we have come to associate
it with health, beauty, sexual vigor and the capacity to cap-
ture something close to permanent youthfulness." In fact,
he argued, the new national preoccupation with weight had
become so all-encompassing that thinness was now part of
the American dream.[1]

The Overweight Society reflected a new focus on bodies and
the need to whittle, shape, and tone them, which consti-

tuted a central part of 1960s culture.[2] The thin body was becoming more important in American culture as a signifier of status, personal style, and beauty. This development allowed the creation of a burgeoning fitness marketplace that included exercise information, instruction, and devices. Whereas federal fitness efforts of the previous decade had attempted to cajole Americans into fitness out of patriotic obligation, new commercial fitness efforts were grounded in the culture of weight reduction and thinness. Exercise as an industry began to flourish as thinness became more fashionable and as physicians began to document excess weight among the American public.

The relationship between weight loss and exercise, however, was a complicated one. Today, these two terms are paired almost unthinkingly in conversation, but in the 1960s, they functioned as separate concepts. Critics often blamed decreasing physical activity for the nation's weight problem, but surprisingly, exercise was not viewed as the solution, especially for women. Rather, dieting was perceived as the best way to lose weight, while exercise was seen primarily as a body toner and shaper. Although the two were imagined differently, over the course of the decade, they worked in concert to increase the cultural significance of the body, with each buttressing interest in the other.

A new exercise media culture sprouted during the last years of the 1950s; Americans began to see exercise shows and commercials for fitness-related products and health clubs on television and viewed news programs that included information about exercise as part of a healthy lifestyle. In music stores, they purchased exercise LPs. In print, they read consumer health guides and instruction manuals that encouraged physical activity and read news about exercise-related research in daily papers and magazines. The evolution in exercise equipment sold in the Sears catalog over the decade is telling: in 1960, exercise merchandise filled a single page; a decade later, fitness-related goods and apparel were featured in several multipage spreads.[3] By 1970, Americans were spending $175 million a year on exercise devices alone.[4]

The increase in exercise wares and services was the result of several influences. The work of the President's Council on Youth Fitness under Eisenhower, discussed in the previous chapter, set the foundation for fitness awareness in the 1950s and helped reveal its profit-making potential to product manufacturers and fitness promoters. The President's Council on Physical Fitness (PCPF) under Kennedy, as well as the president's own example, continued this work, adding nationwide school fitness testing and enlarging the scope of federal fitness promotion for both adults and children.[5] The renamed council reflected a growing interest in physical development not just for youth but for people of all ages. In a direct contradiction of the policy of former director Shane MacCarthy, the reorganized PCPF set absolute physical fitness standards, even though it recognized that only 10 percent of American youth could meet them.[6] American children continued to fail fitness tests throughout the 1960s, but governmental efforts relaxed as alarm gave way to problem solving and popular interest in exercise increased. In 1961, the *Public Relations Journal* noted that the youth fitness message "has found a new market. It has come from the narrow confines of the gymnasium and playing fields to seek, and find, greener pastures on Main Street—not to mention Madison and Fifth Avenues," making it clear that the future of fitness lay not in governmental promotion but in consumer culture.[7]

The transformation of exercise into a popular leisure activity was also the result of a number of expansive alterations in American lifestyles. The postwar economic boom and the changes it enabled, including suburban development, increased automobile ownership, and a number of dietary modifications, contributed significantly to the interest in exercise. At the same time, television, film, fashion, and style icons helped glamorize the "active lifestyle" and normalize the increasingly uncovered body. This combination of changes created a context for the proliferation of exercise even as its definition remained vague and its benefits unclear.

This chapter explores the flowering of commercial exercise culture in the mid-twentieth century, with a focus on exercise promotion directed at women. For women, an exercise routine was part of a beauty regimen, a tool to shape and firm the body. That exercise could contribute to one's health was a concept largely reserved for men (covered in the next chapter). The media became a prolific source of exercise information and helped advance the notion that all women should engage in exercise for beauty and to ensure the longevity of their marriages. By 1969, fitness expert Olga Ley voiced the feelings of many Americans when she admitted, "Today's preoccupation with physical fitness may make a woman feel guilty if she doesn't set aside a special time for exercise."[8] Thus, by the end of the decade, exercise—however one defined it—had become an item on many women's daily to-do lists.

"OUR MODERN WAY OF LIFE"

In the 1950s, members of the President's Council on Youth Fitness had expressed concern about the future of the nation's military. Weak children would make poor soldiers. Their rhetoric, however, was typically limited to the "softening" of young Americans. Only rarely did they express specific concerns about weight: "softness" usually denoted weakness rather than corpulence. This was the case for the national media as well, but as the discussion shifted from the physical capabilities of soldiers to the state of citizens' bodies, the conversation became increasingly oriented toward weight.

In 1952, W. Henry Sebrell Jr., director of the National Institutes of Health, labeled obesity "the nation's top nutritional problem." He estimated that about 25 percent of all Americans were overweight and singled out older women as a special concern, suggesting that as many as 60 percent were obese.[9] Sebrell's pronouncement marked the unofficial start of a new, intense focus on body size and its relationship to health and aesthetics. Americans, it seemed, had never been so fat. Studies, surveys, and polls that measured the number of overweight Americans increased, as did physician interest in the etiology of overweight and its prevention.[10] For instance, the National Health Examination Survey, a widely referenced research project conducted by the federal government from 1960 to 1962, found that about one-quarter of all adults in the United States were overweight. This figure held true for both white and black men and for younger white women; rates were significantly higher for black women and for white women over age fifty.[11]

Making claims about absolute weight gain over time is notoriously difficult, especially when such comparisons rely on studies based on different criteria. Researchers were not always precise, sometimes varying the ways they measured weight or how they defined terms such as *overweight* and *obese*, and they often depended on unreliable subject-supplied data. Moreover, studies often failed to include Americans of color, leading to an incomplete understanding of national trends. Calculating exactly how much weight Americans were gaining was difficult, but the sheer number of studies concluding that Americans were getting larger was hard to ignore.[12] Metropolitan Life weight tables, for instance, reported steady gains between 1941 and 1963, although the increases were stated in pounds rather than percentages.[13] Absolute indicators, such as the need to widen stadium seats, also showed that weight gain was occurring.[14] It seems safe to conclude that some weight gain occurred in the population as a whole between 1945 and 1965, but it is unlikely that researchers will ever be able to document precise increases; the relatively new nature of the problem meant that sophisticated epidemiological tools, along with discipline-wide standards and definitions, had yet to be established.

Experts were not the only ones concerned about Americans' weight; public perception of the problem also seemed to be growing. Network television produced a number of specials focusing on weight and fitness. In 1961, ABC aired *The Flabby American*, which told the story of the nation's unfitness and offered suggestions for improvement.[15] CBS responded a year later with *CBS Reports: The Fat American*, which informed viewers that one in three Americans was overweight.[16] Journalist Howard K. Smith took up the same topic on ABC in his 1962 report *America the Lazy*, featuring TV fitness instructor Debbie Drake; Charles Atlas, creator of the Dynamic Tension mail-order bodybuilding course; gym impresario Vic Tanny; and University of Oklahoma football coach Bud Wilkinson, Kennedy's fitness council director.[17]

Many Americans blamed the country's growing girth on a better standard of living, which was reflected in new trends in housing and lifestyle that reduced physical activity. Commentators of the time usually referred to these changes as "our modern way of life," taking into account not only new housing developments but also the new appliances and machines that filled those houses and the cars necessitated by them. This conversation represented the continuation of a critique of consumption grounded in the physical body that the Kraus-Weber fitness tests had brought to national attention in 1954. But in the 1960s, cars, televisions, appliances, and even single-story ranch houses were blamed not for weakness but for fatness and inactivity. "If Americans now wanted to get exercise," *Good Housekeeping* pointed out in 1963, "[it] must be planned, since it is no longer part of our mechanized existence."[18]

The expansion of the suburbs after World War II was a process enabled by lower home prices, pent-up demand resulting from wartime shortages, special-offer mortgages for returning GIs, and an expanding middle class. Between 1950 and 1960, the suburban population rose from 21 million to 37 million.[19] The idea of suburban living was not new—it had existed since the 1920s—but in previous decades, home builders had followed the patterns of rail and trolley lines, which allowed residents to rely on public transportation. After the war, this was no longer the case; growing car ownership meant that new suburban developments could be built anywhere.[20] As historian Mark S. Foster has observed, "Virtually everything about the new suburbs assumed automobile ownership."[21] Because developers built in areas where land was cheap rather than near conveniences, car travel was required for almost all needs.[22] Reliance on the car meant the end of walking and using public transit for errands, shopping, and commuting. Critics of the new automobility often lamented the death of walking and cited "riding" as a challenge to fitness. Fitness advocate Bonnie Prudden pointed out that the "tyranny of the wheel" began in childhood with the stroller, continued with the school bus, and then moved to the car.[23] Mothers' new role as the family chauffeur and expanding car ownership among teenagers were also cited as evidence that Americans were engaging in less physical activity.

Although the suburbs were often portrayed as an ideal location to raise a family, children were thought to be in particular danger as new suburban lifestyles changed patterns of physical activity. Critics argued that children had better access to parks and playgrounds in urban areas and lamented the clearing of trees for housing developments.[24] School districts in the new suburbs were particularly challenged by the number of baby-boom children, and they had difficulty providing adequate facilities.[25] In 1957, for example, 91 percent of the nation's elementary schools lacked gymnasiums.[26] In the wake of *Sputnik*, some school authorities argued that funds were better spent on science and math education rather than expensive athletic facilities.[27]

It should be noted that the sweeping changes of the new suburbia excluded a large segment of the population: African Americans were often unable to take advantage of government-backed mortgages because integrated areas were considered poor credit risks.[28] Moreover, even if funds were available, restrictive covenants in new suburban developments typically limited home ownership to whites only. Prior to 1960, African Americans constituted only 5 percent of the suburban population; after that time, the black suburban population grew to about 2.5 million residents, typically in all-black enclaves or on the West Coast.[29]

The same dramatic changes that impacted Americans' physical activity were also affecting their eating habits. At the same 1952 meeting of the National Food and Nutrition Institute where Sebrell declared obesity a concern, his colleague from the Bureau of Agricultural Economics, Frederick V. Waugh, reported that per capita food consumption in the United States had increased by 12 percent. Consumption of more costly foods such as meat, eggs, citrus fruits, and tomatoes was on the rise, while the consumption of potatoes had declined.[30] Waugh's report reflected the eating climate of the postwar years. After the privations of the Depression and rationing during World War II, hearty eating habits and the consumption of premium foods signaled a return to normalcy. The booming postwar economy, which had enriched and enlarged the middle class, meant that more people were able to enjoy more expensive foods. According to food historians Jane and Michael Stern, it was during the 1950s and 1960s that Americans "fell in love with deluxe food, vintage wine and the joy of cooking."[31] A "gourmet" movement, inspired by televised cooking shows, transatlantic travel, and returned GIs, ushered in an era of exuberant cuisine that tended toward large portions, exotic ingredients, heavy sauces, and dramatic flair.[32] Food-related social activities became a cornerstone of suburban life. Barbecues, made possible by backyards, grew in popularity and gave men the opportunity to cook.[33] Social drinking and cocktail hours became a regular part of neighborhood social life. Liquor manufacturers promoted the consumption of high-calorie alcohol as a mark of sophisticated taste and, for men, of masculinity.[34] During the decade of the 1960s, food consumption increased even as household food expenditures decreased. According to Wyden, on average, 22.5 percent of the family budget was spent on food in 1963, versus 28.4 percent in 1953.[35] At the same time, consumption of premium goods, such as beef and sugar, also increased.[36] Larger kitchens in suburban homes also allowed more food storage. Sizable home freezers, along with the ease of transporting large quantities of food thanks to automobiles, led to the idea that pantries should always be full and cold storage always stocked.[37]

In addition to growing portion sizes and richer ingredients, larders were increasingly filled with processed convenience foods. Corporations began to play a larger role in setting American tables at midcentury. Innovations in food chemistry created 400 food additives between 1949 and 1959; this led to the development of new food products, many of dubious nutritional value, such as TV dinners, processed cheese, and freeze-dried potato flakes.[38] Manufacturers provided back-of-the-box recipes, creative advertising, and their own cookbooks to teach home cooks how to use unfamiliar products. Although some of this chemical prowess was evident in the creation of new diet foods and drinks, advertisers were also working to maximize opportunities for consumption through snacking. The Lipton Soup Company, for example, made California dip a party staple in 1954 with the invention of its freeze-dried onion soup mix and its back-of-the-box recipe.[39] And between 1950 and 1960, potato chip production in the United States nearly doubled.[40] Snacking was increasingly associated with television and film viewing, and some new snack foods were marketed specifically to children, who, as many women's magazines noted, were increasingly overweight.[41] Frito-Lay, for example, used the cartoon characters the Frito Kid and the Frito Bandito to sell its corn chips in the 1960s.[42]

Americans were also eating out more often. The 1960s became "the age of the suburban coffee shop," with new chains opening and expanding rapidly. Fast-food restaurants, which had existed since the 1920s, were becoming an increasingly important segment of the restaurant scene as harried suburban mothers chauffeured hungry children to after-school activities.[43] By 1963, $19 billion was spent on meals eaten away from home, an increase of $8 billion since 1950.[44] "There is no way of estimating how many tons of excess weight are being added to the American waistline by the pizza parlor or by that more modern institution, the Pancake House, with its dozens of varieties," Wyden complained in *The Overweight Society*.[45]

These changes in food consumption habits, combined with less physical activity in Americans' daily lives, took their toll on their bodies. Stanley Garn, a child development expert who participated in the 1960 White House Conference on Children and Youth, summed up the new environment, whose effects were not limited to children:

> Through the stimulation of advertising tap water is being replaced by sugared juices, milk and carbonated drinks. Snacks have become a ritualized part of the movies and are inseparably associated with television viewing. Avenues for caloric expenditure are gradually diminishing. . . . As suburbia expands into the denuded suburbs, there are fewer trees to climb, fewer things to do. The car-pool and the school-bus reduce the energy expenditure and the ranch house no longer provides calorie-expending stairs to climb.[46]

Yet, even as Americans were becoming heavier, the importance of thinness in American culture was growing. Thinness had been an important fashion trend for American women since the turn of the century. The Gibson girl, flappers, and actress Clara Bow had gradually introduced the idea of thinness as a fashion statement in the early years of the twentieth century, but as historian Roberta Pollack Seid notes, the standard was not monolithic and could vary, depending on a woman's age.[47] Over time, the acceptable range for women's figures began to narrow. Women's clothes in the immediate postwar era, for example, emphasized a trim waistline as part of fashion designer Christian Dior's influential "New Look," causing industry insiders to wonder "where we would get models who could fit into them."[48] In the 1950s, however, these fashion ideals still coexisted with voluptuous film stars such as Marilyn Monroe and Jane Russell, who provided an alternative model of feminine beauty. In 1953, Gallup polls indicated that slightly more women wanted to remain their current size or gain weight (52 percent) than wanted to reduce (42 percent).[49] But as the decade progressed, thin became the only ideal body type for American women. Seid identifies 1958 as a critical year, when fashion magazine *Vogue* began to pay more attention to the shape and size of models' bodies than to the clothing they wore.[50] Karal Ann Marling argues that the trend toward thinness occurred slightly later, when fashion shifted from the New Look—which, in addition to a pinched waist called for full skirts and even padding to "accentuate the swelling of the hips"—to the "sack," a shapeless shift that became popular in the early 1960s.[51] For historian Lois Banner, celebrity models such as Suzy Parker and Twiggy and the growing interest in fashion photography in the early 1960s were responsible for the ascendance of thinness.[52]

Clearly, all these trends played a role in intensifying the preference for thinness among high-fashion authorities. Nevertheless, its rise as the most important signifier of a woman's beauty seemed to surprise some, prompting Ladies' Home Journal to observe in 1961 that, "rather suddenly we became a weight conscious nation."[53] Whereas in the past clothing had been an ally in hiding "figure faults" and "sloppy posture," it was now a foe, with revealing cuts and shorter hemlines emphasizing the body more than the garments. Jean Noe, a syndicated writer for the Women's News Service, told her readers in 1966 that in order to wear the season's new clothes, their bodies would have to adapt, but obtaining the proper physique would not be that simple. She encouraged women to "take your vitamins, join the health club, drink no-cal soft drinks, exercise with weights, drink Metrecal for lunch, eat yogurt, stop smoking, don't bite your nails and don't eat fried foods. If you do all this, plus more, you'll possibly be able to pass the test to wear spring's new clothes—clothes that seem to make the body beneath them almost as important as the clothes themselves."[54] Viewed within a history of female body shape, these comments suggest that thinness had become both more extreme and totalizing; the body was no longer viewed as a fixed entity but as a malleable accessory, adaptable to its possessor's latest whim.

There were a few exceptions to these trends, however. The African American community, for example, did not accord the same importance to weight loss that white Americans did. Black newspapers such as the Baltimore Afro-American and the Chicago Defender occasionally published articles on weight loss for health or beauty, but much less often than other papers did. Historian Carolyn de la Pena rightly draws attention to the fact that characterizations of American aesthetic preferences have typically excluded African Americans. Historically, beauty trends among women of color have been more focused on hair products and cosmetics than on thinness.[55] Peter Stearns has shown that in the African American community, the positive association between strength and size, the religious notion of a God-given body, and male preferences for larger women have allowed a wider range of acceptable body types.[56]

Concerns about weight were not entirely absent from black women's minds, even if they were not preoccupied with extreme thinness. Era Bell Thompson, for example, wrote about her weight loss travails for Ebony in 1968, notably focusing on the health benefits of a thinner figure rather than on appearance. "Big Fat Mama may be fun to sing about, but unless she changes her eating habits her days are numbered," Thompson wrote, pointing out that half of all middle-aged black women were overweight and that hypertension and diabetes occurred at significantly higher rates in blacks than in whites. In the African American community, according to Thompson's physician, awareness of the dangers of obesity increased in conjunction with education and professional status. Citing diet pills, fad diets, hypnosis, weight-loss surgery, and health spas (which, wrote Thompson, "Neither can I afford, nor would I likely be accepted by"), she demonstrated a familiarity with the same weight-loss techniques featured in white women's magazines. Rejecting exercise and embracing calorie counting, Thompson declared, "For my own sake I want to reduce." Appropriating the language of the civil rights movement but, at the same time, nodding to African American beauty concerns, she announced, "Now, I have the will power. With my 'good' hair and beautiful color, I shall overcome."[57] Thompson's article is evidence that, by the late 1960s, interest in weight reduction was growing in the African American community. This convergence of black and white beauty concerns was also demonstrated by the inroads made by African American models in the fashion industry, whose lithe bodies were just as thin as white models'.[58]

GLAMORIZING THE ACTIVE LIFESTYLE

Along with fears of corpulence, thinness as a fashion style and the notion of the body as an accessory helped generate interest in exercise. In addition to these trends, two other developments were raising the profile of exercise as a leisure activity and, at the same time, further normalizing the increasingly bare physique: the popularity of "California living" and the example set by a young, physically active president.

In the 1960s, Americans became enamored of television shows, films, and music centered on California beach life. The warm-weather sporting activities associated with sun and surf, such as boating, waterskiing, and surfing, highlighted the place of the body in popular culture and drew attention to physical activity.[59] Media depictions of California living showed that a young, fit body was both necessary for and the result of life in the sun. Throughout the decade, beaches were a popular backdrop for films and television shows. Surfing ingenue Gidget, played by Sandra Dee in the movies and Sally Field on television, popularized beach life in Southern California.[60] The young, suntanned stars were most often clad in swim attire. In the original film, waif-like Sandra Dee models no fewer than five bathing suits. American International Pictures took advantage of the interest in California to produce a series of very popular low-budget beach movies. With titles such as *Muscle Beach Party* (which combines a surf theme with a parody of Muscle Beach in Venice, California) and *How to Stuff a Wild Bikini*, these movies made it clear that having a trim, healthy body was part of the California fantasy.[61]

The California lifestyle was transformed into a physical aesthetic: thin, tan, taut bodies with sun-bleached blond hair and pearly white teeth. Women's magazines showed readers how to create the Golden State look at home through hairstyling, makeup, and fashion.[62] The preoccupation with California living also inspired cosmetics lines and advertising campaigns. Products such as Cutex nail polish and Tampax tampons referenced the California scene in ads featuring active young women on sandy landscapes. Just lounging on the beach was no longer enough; as Tampax saw it, young women of the 1960s surfed, rode motorcycles, scuba dived, and water-skied.[63] In 1966, writer Gael Greene profiled an apartment complex near Los Angeles that catered to young singles by providing a full complement of group activities and the latest amenities, including two swimming pools, a whirlpool, three tennis courts, two gyms, and two saunas. The "new way of life in California" meant that the revealed, active body was at the center of one's social calendar. The focus of Greene's article, a twenty-five-year-old transplanted midwesterner named Jan, told about sending her one-piece bathing suit "home to my mother because boys kept asking why I was wearing that baggy suit," illustrating that covering up one's figure was no longer an option.[64]

On the East Coast, a complementary trend was unfolding. The election of the nation's first celebrity president in 1960 drew attention to the leisure activities of the upper class. Photos of the Kennedy clan playing football, sailing, golfing, and enjoying the outdoors circulated widely, making it clear that "vigah," vitality, and healthy bodies were the result of a life lived fully. Articles discussing the fitness promotion efforts of the new administration almost always mentioned the president's own example.[65] In 1964, GQ noted that "exercise is 'in'" and credited the late president "with creating the glowing new image of physical fitness through vigorous activity." The magazine observed, "No longer does reference to exercise bring to mind a ninety-pound weakling straining at barbells," hinting at an obviously distasteful, working-class Charles Atlas. "The President changed this, for he was . . . often photographed swimming, golfing, sailing before breakfast or choosing up sides for a touch football game between lunch and dinner."[66] Jackie Kennedy set the same example for women. One newsmagazine called the First Lady the "most athletic wife of a president in memory," and photographs of her riding horses, swimming, and water-skiing appeared in national publications.[67] The Kennedy example made healthy bodies seem like a natural extension of the "good life" and bestowed an aura of sophistication on physical activity. While waterskiing and touch football were quite different from the calisthenics routines prescribed by fitness proponents, the attractive glow they cast helped make exercise not just a necessary activity (for thinness or weight reduction) but desirable as well. Actors in beach movies and members of the Kennedy clan seemed to be having fun, and their sporty, trim bodies were an integral part of that enjoyment.

EXERCISE ADVICE FOR AMERICAN WOMEN

These multiple contexts, along with the promotional efforts of exercise entrepreneurs, led to considerable interest in exercise for thinness and style, even though dieting was considered a more effective way to shed pounds.

Although discussions of obesity had framed it as a national health issue, most articles offering specific solutions focused on women's appearance rather than their health. Women's magazines were rife with meal plans and weight-loss success stories.[68] Low-calorie cookbooks exploded in popularity, and diet books hit the best-seller lists.[69] As one exercise book noted, "To be 'with it' today, you have to diet. People who know virtually nothing about food, know all about diets: low cholesterol, high protein, crash, liquid, banana, steak, cheese, all-meat, cooked, raw, ten-day, thirty-day, pills, tablets, wafers, all-fluid, no-fluid, mush."[70] Reacting to the seemingly endless discussions of weight reduction, one magazine columnist exclaimed, "If you're on a diet, shut up!"[71]

Many of the popular weight-loss plans of the 1960s would be considered extreme by today's standards, with some of the more restrictive ones limiting dieters to 800 calories a day.[72] Sales of diet drinks and appetite suppressants totaled $170 million in 1961, already four times the amount spent on these products in 1958.[73] National retailer Sears Roebuck sold a full complement of capsules, weight-loss gum, and appetite-suppressant "candy" in its semiannual catalog.[74] And at least one laxative marketed itself as a weight-loss aid.[75] If a dieter wasn't successful on her own, she could turn to one of several newly established group programs. Overeaters Anonymous was established in 1960, followed by Weight Watchers a year later. Both of these followed TOPS (Taking Off Pounds Sensibly), founded in 1948.[76]

The role of exercise in weight loss was not entirely clear to women of the 1960s. For laypersons, questions about how to define exercise, how long to perform it, and how effective it was would not be resolved until the end of the decade. During these years, numerous authorities with diverse viewpoints would emerge to create awareness of but also confusion about exercise, leaving most women to decide for themselves whether a particular program, instructor, or device was effective. Although TV exercise-show hosts, instruction manuals, and even some physicians recommended exercise for general well-being and sometimes for weight loss, there was tremendous doubt about its usefulness. Article titles such as "Shape up and Slim Down (with 68 Diet Tips and Eight Lazy Exercises)" illustrate the importance of dieting in relation to exercise.[77] *Redbook*, for example, told

readers, "If you're exercising just because you think you should, forget it;
you probably won't keep it up, and your muscles won't get much out of
it."[78] *Weight Watchers Magazine* told readers in its inaugural issue in 1968
that if they weren't exercising before beginning their dieting efforts, there
was no reason to start—instead, they should wait to exercise until *after* they
had lost weight, so they would look more attractive in a leotard.[79]

Many laypeople and physicians believed that exercise was in fact detrimental to weight-loss efforts because it induced hunger.[80] Others argued
that the amount of exercise needed to burn off even a single meal was so
high as to render the activity useless. "Exercise? I have nothing against
exercise, but it's hard to imagine a more inefficient way to lose weight,"
one physician scoffed.[81] Drs. Philip Gelvin and Thomas McGavack, who
directed the obesity clinic at Metropolitan Hospital in New York, were similarly doubtful. Citing time constraints, increased appetite, and possible
health risks, they observed, "Of course, hard physical labor can result in a
tremendous energy output . . . but how practical is this as a common procedure to effect weight reduction?"[82] Even those physicians who thought
exercise might be useful to maintain one's current weight agreed that
it was simply too much work for too little return. Dr. Seymour Halpern
told readers of one women's magazine that "exercise should not be depended on as a method of weight loss—you'd have to exercise too much,"
although he admitted it was "a reasonable way to prevent weight gain."[83]
To counter these beliefs, pro-exercise medical authorities, such as Harvard
nutritionist Jean Mayer and physician Paul Dudley White, felt the need to
defend it publicly.[84] The publication of instructional exercise spreads in
many of the same magazines that cast doubt on exercise's benefits undoubtedly created confusion for readers.

It's easy to see why exercise was not viewed as a weight-loss technique,
given the sedateness of most of the programs outlined in instruction
manuals and women's magazines. Most of them defined exercise as a series of calisthenics or "setting up exercises" that included arm circles, toe
touches, waist twisting, and leg lifts. For women, the emphasis was on
graceful, balletic, nonstrenuous movements. On most exercise records,
the accompanying music tended toward orchestral arrangements with
gentle, flowing melodies.[85] It would be another decade before jogging

redefined exercise as necessarily strenuous and made it socially acceptable for women to perspire. Thus, women in the 1960s were counseled to
"always relax before repeating an exercise" and to "stop before you start
to feel tired."[86] *Redbook*'s "Secret Workout" outlined a series of isometric
exercises that women could do while having a drink at a cocktail party or
toweling off after a shower.[87] One suggested plan in *Good Housekeeping* told
readers to exercise on their beds after lunch.[88] Another *Good Housekeeping*
article pointed out that "exhausting calisthenics" were inappropriate for
the female body and recommended "a series of rhythmic movements, done
with controlled deep breathing, that leaves you relaxed and rejuvenated."[89]
The idea that exercise didn't need to be strenuous also helps explain the
vigorous sales of electrical massagers and stimulators, body rollers, and
steam cabinets during the decade.[90] Given the working definition of exercise simply as purposeful movements, it seems reasonable for Americans
to assume that such devices would be just as effective as exercise.

While the value of exercise as a calorie-burning activity was debatable,
most sources agreed that it was useful for shaping and toning the body.
Promoters argued that in addition to functioning as a beauty technique,
exercise could create a happier matrimonial relationship, based on the
premise that a woman's worth as a marriage partner depended in large part
on her appearance. Popular television exercise-show host Debbie Drake
made it clear that a shapely figure was the key to a good marriage when
she titled her 1964 exercise record *How to Keep Your Husband Happy: Look
Slim! Keep Trim! Exercise along with Debbie Drake.* The album's cover depicted
a thoughtful, reclining man in an aqua sweater vest with the leotard-clad
Drake kicking and stretching in his thoughts (illustrated by a bubble).[91]
The back cover asked, "Do you know that overweight is a threat to the
happiest of marriages? The obese wife knows she is a disappointment to
her husband. It is dangerous to family contentment and security when
Mamma is the best advertisement for her own calorie-burdened cooking.
Fighting against weight is one of the surest ways of fighting for husband's
continued love, and getting it."[92] It then broke down the female body into
component parts, with information on how each should be maintained so
as to retain a husband's attention. Drake also provided a helpful checklist
of fourteen tips "for keeping your husband happy," including "1. Firm and

graceful body. . . . 8. Excess fat (taboo)."[93] Drake made no reference to a woman's health. Rather, exercise was a way for a wife to demonstrate her love for her husband by maintaining her body.

After children entered the picture, women were still held to a thin ideal. Even Bonnie Prudden, who espoused a no-nonsense approach to exercise for all, seemed to embrace the notion that women needed to stay slim to remain attractive to their husbands. Her after-thirty exercise guide related one obstetrician's tendency to castigate mothers when they were slow to lose weight after delivering. As Prudden saw it, "This young doctor was taking care of that baby's future as well as its prenatal life. Whether he knew it or not, and I always thought he did, he was taking a strong interest in the happiness of the baby's father, as well as its mother."[94] For Prudden, a shapely figure was a marriage requirement long after the wedding.

Advertisements also informed women that staying trim was a necessary part of marriage. Ads for Sego liquid meal replacement, for example, made it clear that the key to matrimonial bliss was an attractive body: "Your honeymoon figure . . . how slender it was. Would he think so now?" one 1963 ad taunted.[95] The manufacturers of Relax-a-Cizor, an electrical toning device, told *Good Housekeeping* readers: "Modern women know that a 'wedding-day' figure means marriage long romance . . . a more confident . . . outlook, [and] the contentment you feel in knowing your family is proud of your appearance."[96] The maker of Ayds weight-loss "candy" employed scare tactics when it mocked up its *Ladies' Home Journal* ad to resemble the magazine's monthly weight-loss narrative: "I live in a hotel. Alone," homemaker Farley Heward lamented. "When my husband married me, I was fairly thin. But when he left me I was fat."[97]

Exercise records, instruction manuals, and magazines had long been the main source of exercise information for women. The invention of television and the subsequent expansion of daytime programming that targeted stay-at-home housewives in the late 1950s introduced a new source of information and increased the presence of exercise in women's lives. Weekday exercise shows introduced the idea that exercise should be a part of women's everyday routine. The shows created a platform for the display of fit and attractive bodies; their hosts made health, appearance, and nutrition a topic of daily conversation, and they increased the diffusion of exercise information exponentially. Television exercise shows also provided a level of instruction that was not possible on radio programs or exercise records. Exercise shows, as well as fitness segments in magazine-format programs, were a logical fit with other fashion and glamour advice that constituted the bulk of early daytime TV programming.[98]

Today, Jack La Lanne may be the only instructor remembered from the first generation of TV exercise shows, but he had numerous colleagues and competitors on local stations and national networks. These programs' long runs, their enthusiastic reception by viewers, the number of presenters, and the notoriety they attracted all attest that a vibrant fitness culture was developing rapidly in the 1960s. Sadly, relatively little footage of these early television exercise shows exists today because they were considered too ephemeral to conserve or because producers reused film (re-recording over previous shows) to save money. This means that scholars have access to many of these programs only through newspaper columns about them, as well as companion books and records. (La Lanne's shows are the only real exception.[99]) Furthermore, television historians have neglected this field of production; episode guides, performer indices, and analytical scholarship have overlooked these shows. It is likely that many more such programs, especially local productions, existed in addition to those discussed here.

Television helped locate exercise as both a form of labor and a form of leisure for American women. Daytime television programmers were initially faced with a dilemma. Unlike radio, which allowed women to attend to household duties while listening, the new visual medium was considered too demanding to permit simultaneous housework and attention to the TV set. Networks struggled to develop new kinds of shows that viewers could follow while doing their chores. As a result, a number of techniques were created to encourage a kind of distracted viewing so that women's work time and leisure time could coincide.[100] Exercise shows represented a disruption of this model, however. On the one hand, to get the benefit of the program, the housewife had to cease her work and focus on herself, making exercise a kind of pleasurable self-care. On the other hand, in the context of household labor and in response to social pressures, exercise could also be perceived as an unavoidable wifely duty.

Just as some programs told viewers when it was important to turn their attention to the screen, Jack La Lanne ("rhymes with pain," as several commentators quipped) typically opened his show by instructing the children who had been watching the preceding program "to run and go get Mother."[101] Once she arrived, La Lanne's white German shepherd Happy was called on to perform a trick for the kids, and Mother was told to put down her work, her coffee, and her cigarettes and to participate in the day's exercises, which he called "trimnastics," hinting at the era's preoccupation with thinness. Although La Lanne occasionally made reference to male viewers, the context of the show, as well as its weekday morning time slot, made it clear that women were his primary audience. La Lanne's backdrop resembled the homes he imagined his viewers resided in: a living room complete with that marker of suburban architecture—a picture window. Accompanied by a live organist, La Lanne's exercises were performed to zippy renditions of traditional tunes such as "A Bicycle Built for Two" and "De Camptown Races." La Lanne used no special equipment other than a Glamour-Stretcher (an elastic rubber cable he sold by mail), a chair, and occasionally a towel or a book (for weight resistance). Abdominal crunches, calf raises, jumping jacks, and many of the movements performed with the Glamour-Stretcher, such as upright rows, are regularly performed in gyms today.[102] Other familiar moves, such as arm circles, toe touches, and running in place, have largely been relegated to the fitness dustbin. La Lanne also had a penchant for hand, face, and neck exercises, which he claimed would firm loose jowls and necklines. These unusual movements, which called for towels and hand pressure against the face for added resistance, were perhaps the least likely to produce results.

La Lanne began his television career in California with a successful local exercise show in 1951. The show went national in 1958, and by 1965, it was broadcast in eighty American cities to an estimated audience of 40 million.[103] La Lanne had no script; he spoke earnestly into the camera, and his frequent speech flubs and "on second thought" routine changes made him seem accessible and natural. Newsweek called the show "a mixture of cornball and wheat germ."[104] During the short program, La Lanne played the roles of personal trainer, cheerleader, and therapist. He regularly lectured on the importance of proper eating, and many of his beliefs—considered odd back then—have stood the test of time. He advocated the consumption of brown rice, fish, wheat germ, cheese, and fruit and the avoidance of white flour and sugar. He often railed against what he called "foodless foods" and junk-food advertisements directed at children.[105] On Thursdays, he prepared recipes in the set's home kitchen, showcasing such dishes as "beauty salad" (a mixed vegetable salad), steamed fish with soy sauce, and stuffed bell peppers with brown rice. La Lanne took pains to make the show enjoyable. Although he disapproved of smoking and excessive coffee and alcohol consumption, he never gave absolute rules, believing that once viewers took up a regular exercise regimen, they would naturally gravitate toward a healthier lifestyle. Exercise, as La Lanne depicted it, was not work but a form of leisure. After a commercial break, he regularly began the new segment by telling viewers, "Let's get back to play."

Certainly, part of the appeal of La Lanne's show was his remarkable body. In an era when few men displayed such well-developed musculature, La Lanne's form-fitting jumpsuit left little to the imagination. His clothing was so tight that sometimes (in this pre-spandex era) he had to unbuckle his waist clasp to perform an exercise. Reportedly sporting measurements of 48-27-34, La Lanne's physical attributes were not lost on viewers.[106] While answering the mail, as he did every Tuesday, he read aloud a letter from one woman who asked why he didn't remove his shirt to exercise. "We would like to see what a real chest would look like, for all we see is the flab of our husbands," she complained. La Lanne, gallant and charming as always, replied that he was privileged to be a guest in the viewer's home and, as such, would not disrobe.[107]

Perhaps La Lanne's enthusiastic, ever-positive, and sympathetic demeanor left viewers wishing that their husbands shared some of his personality characteristics as well. His five-day schedule made him a fixture in women's lives and provided the basis for an emotional connection, which La Lanne worked to promote. He suggestively reminded viewers, "We have a date every day." He regularly told the audience how much this time with "his students" meant to him and how much he looked forward to their next session, and he always thanked them for allowing him into their homes. Often La Lanne's shows ended with him serenading viewers in a lovely tenor, crooning, "I'm going to be missing you wherever you are."[108] His

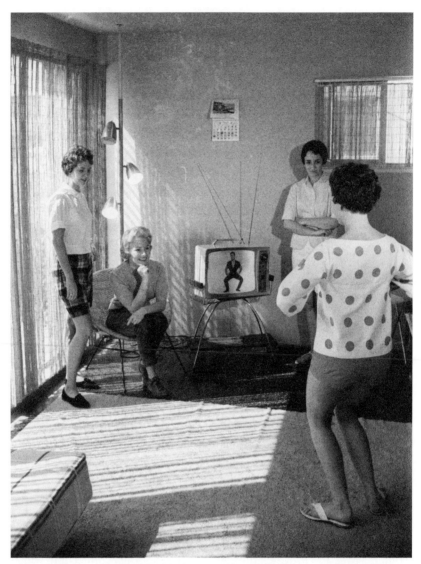

Television offered a new source of health, fitness, and beauty information, particularly for midcentury housewives. Exercise shows, which were typically broadcast during the hours women were doing their household chores, located fitness as a form of both leisure and labor. Women sometimes gathered in one another's homes and exercised together, as shown in this 1960 photo taken in Southern California. (© Roxann Livingston. Photograph by Earl Theisen, Look Magazine Photograph Collection, Prints and Photographs Division, Library of Congress, LC Job 60-4468-5-Frame 24)

habit of calling out encouragement to viewers by name not only deepened his relationship with fans but also encouraged them to write in for airtime recognition and join a community of exercisers. Some viewer letters indicated that women gathered to watch and exercise in groups at home. According to one report, La Lanne received 1,000 fan letters a day.[109]

La Lanne's allure made him fit for membership in a group of men *Time* dubbed the "charm boys." Though the magazine referred to game and variety show hosts such as Garry Moore, Arthur Godfrey, and Art Linkletter, La Lanne could also be included. As Marsha Cassidy argues in her study of women's daytime television viewing, these male hosts "woo[ed] the homemaker with an appealing but low-key sexuality." These men's daily presence in viewers' lives, in the absence of their husbands, created an "illusion of closeness" and companionship and imparted "a discrete sensuality to a viewer's day."[110] The combination of La Lanne's kindness, his enthusiasm, and his attractive form made him irresistible. *Sports Illustrated* picked up on La Lanne's charm, warning the magazine's presumably male readership of the "consciously seductive man in middle age [who] steps across a Hollywood stage and projects himself—almost bodily—into the home of the beholder, his arms outstretched as if to embrace her."[111]

Other male exercise instructors imitated La Lanne's style. *Ed Allen Time* ran on Chicago and Detroit stations five days a week in the 1960s. In Detroit, three out of four television sets were tuned in to the 9:30 show at various periods during the decade.[112] Resembling Jack La Lanne in appeal and physique, the Canadian Allen made no secret of his measurements (45-31-39), which he showed off in a skin-tight T-shirt and close-fitting slacks. One wife quipped that she got back at her Debbie Drake–loving husband by watching Allen, although she also got a workout: "I do more than exercise my eyeballs."[113] Allen reportedly received 3,000 fan letters a week.[114]

Some male instructors were accompanied by an attractive model-cum-student, replicating the atmosphere of an exercise class. The model allowed the instructor to more fully explain the exercise movements; she also provided inspiration for female audience members and perhaps visual interest for the occasional male viewer. Richard Hittleman's show *Yoga for Health* went on the air in Los Angeles in 1961 to compete with La Lanne. As Hittleman explained the poses, his wife Diane demonstrated

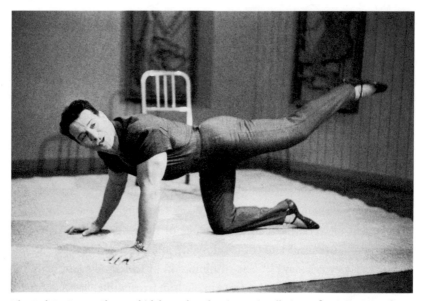

The Jack La Lanne Show, which began broadcasting nationally in 1958, was just one of many TV exercise shows aimed at housewives. La Lanne's peppy and supportive demeanor made him an instant celebrity, and his exceptional physique was not lost on viewers. One fan suggested that he remove his shirt to exercise, complaining, "We would like to see what a real chest would look like for all we see is the flab of our husbands." (© Roxann Livingston. Photograph by Earl Theisen, Look Magazine Photograph Collection, Prints and Photographs Division, Library of Congress, LC Job 60-4468-7-Frame 31)

them, clad in a leotard and fishnet stockings. Diane was never identified as Hittleman's wife, "on the theory that a little mystery about a beautiful girl won't hurt sales."[115] Hittleman sold booklets describing the yoga poses on his show for a dollar; in the first month alone, he claimed to have received 14,000 requests.[116]

Paul Fogarty made use of a former Miss Chicago to demonstrate exercises as he performed the role of instructor. Fogarty transitioned his radio show Keep Fit to Music to television in 1950 with Your Figure, Ladies on Chicago's WGN.[117] Rather than his body, critics commented on Fogarty's breezy manner and quick wit. Like La Lanne, Fogarty imagined himself in women's homes, telling the children to "keep an eye on Mamma" and warning viewers not to kick the cocker spaniel while exercising.[118] The show was so popular that when it went off the air for nine months, viewer demand brought it back.[119]

Hosts with positive, upbeat messages were more successful than those who employed fear or a sense of obligation. Debbie Drake warned that wives who neglected their appearance were in danger of losing their husbands, and she advised women who had difficulty getting motivated to "strip down and have a look in the mirror."[120] Drake's message echoed women's magazines and diet-food advertisers that claimed a successful marriage was dependent on the wife's appearance. Unlike La Lanne, who was both an object of attraction and a confidant, Drake seemed to represent both the figure viewers hoped to attain if they followed her program and the threat of the "other woman" if they did not. Drake's popularity was intense but relatively short-lived. After hosting local programs in Dayton and Indianapolis, her show went into national syndication in 1961. She also penned a newspaper column ("Date with Debbie") carried by sixty papers, recorded two exercise albums, and published three exercise books.[121] Her self-titled television show ran until 1964. During the years she was in the public eye, Drake enjoyed a measure of celebrity, making appearances on talk shows and even inspiring Sears to sell a Debbie Drake doll in 1963.[122]

Press reports never failed to point out her 115-pound figure and measurements of $38\frac{1}{2}$-$22\frac{1}{2}$-36.[123] The form-fitting leotard she wore, as well as the fact that some stations broadcast her show at odd hours, meant that her audience extended beyond those interested in exercise. A letter writer in Chicago confided to an advice columnist that her husband "won't come to dinner until the show's over. . . . The food's chilling, I'm burning, and he's drooling," she complained.[124] One Los Angeles housewife similarly grumbled that KTLA's airing of the series at midnight could only be intended as a "cheap burlesque show."[125] Time seemed to agree that much of Drake's popularity was due to her appearance, noting, "It is hard to roll about on the floor and at the same time watch Debbie with the concentration she deserves."[126]

Despite Drake's successful use of her sex appeal, other female fitness instructors did not follow suit. Typically, female instructors on TV highlighted what they had in common with their viewers at home. For example, a woman's success in regaining her figure after childbirth was frequently mentioned in promotional literature; this not only created a bond between instructor and viewer but also demonstrated the effectiveness of the exercise routine. Margaret Firth's *It's Fun to Reduce* aired five mornings a week on the DuMont network in Pittsburgh and eventually expanded to syndication. Unlike most self-taught exercise entrepreneurs, Firth had a degree in physical education.[127] Mentions of her show in the press always commented on her figure and her four children.[128] *Exercise with Gloria*, hosted by Gloria Roeder, went on the air in 1964 and ran until the end of the decade. Her six daughters were regulars on the show, exercising along with her; the family also appeared on her album *Exercise with Gloria and Her Six Daughters for Family Fitness Fun.*[129] Although Bonnie Prudden was one of the best-known exercise instructors of the 1960s, she did not star in her own show until 1968. Prudden had established a reputation as a fitness authority with the creation of the President's Council on Youth Fitness in the mid-1950s, but her impatience with government bureaucracy soon put her at odds with its leadership. Publicly, she said of the council, "a greater stupidity there never was." Prudden revamped her fitness efforts, producing exercise programs for magazine articles, her own books, and LPs and making regular appearances on other TV shows, including *Today* and *Arthur Godfrey Time.*[130]

The amount of viewer mail received by many of these instructors indicates the degree to which women responded to the exercise genre. The fact that viewers gathered to exercise in groups suggests that they derived a certain enjoyment from the shows—if not from the exercise, then from the companionship. Although magazines often depicted exercise as a chore to be avoided, letters from Margaret Firth's viewers frequently expressed their enjoyment of the program and the exercises. A fan from Woodland Hills, California, began exercising along with the show on the advice of her physician, whose own wife had recommended the program. "I set about it grimly at first," she admitted, "but now I look forward to it as a part of the day's occupations." Her word choice indicates a sense of both enjoyment and duty, which was likely similar to other women's experiences.[131]

Exercise instruction in the early 1960s began to lengthen the list of benefits exercise was said to provide. In addition to an improved figure, some exercisers might take up a routine in the hope that a few toe touches and arm circles would give them more energy or a more charismatic personality. Magazines and television presenters frequently pointed out that in addition to reshaping a woman's body, exercise could increase her energy level and even help her develop a more personable disposition. *Ladies' Home Journal*, for example, likened exercise to sleep, advising tired women, "The next time you feel sluggish or tense pass up the pep pill or tranquilizer and take exercise."[132] In 1960, the Equitable Life Assurance Society gave away free exercise booklets written by Bonnie Prudden for a promotion entitled "How to Find More Energy!" The booklet depicted a mother in the kitchen doing knee bends while father and daughter looked on from the dining room. The photo seemed to suggest that a few extra exercises might supply the homemaker with the energy needed to keep up with her never-ending household chores.[133] Even though women were being told that the task of keeping house was less taxing than ever before, thanks to washing machines, dishwashers, and other kitchen conveniences, it's unlikely they felt this way. In the 1950s and 1960s, the demands of caring for a home, husband, and children were substantial. Time saved by new gadgets was quickly absorbed by school, church, and community activities and increased standards of cleanliness.[134]

If continued attention to the well-being of others left a woman unfulfilled, exercise could be the solution. Exercise promoters regularly suggested that an energetic spirit—the result of a regular fitness regimen—would lead to a more dynamic and pleasant personality. In short, exercisers would become happier people. The therapeutic ethos was a growing part of exercise culture. On television, shows such as *Queen for a Day* and *Glamour Girl* had already situated the physical transformation as the crucial beginning of a total life makeover.[135] Exercise guides similarly promoted the notion that physical changes led to an improved mental outlook. The author of *A Better Figure for You*, for example, linked a fit body with a jovial disposition: "The physically fit person believes that health is one of life's greatest values. She is buoyant, happy, attractive and fun to be around."[136] In slightly more metaphysical prose, *Feel Fine, Look Lovely* informed readers that improved physical fitness would create mental well-being and a charismatic nature. "Confidence of physical grace gives emotional ease," the author promised. "Good looks are enhanced by the entire system being in 'tone,' and therefore, in tune with itself. As the ability to move easily and endurance increase, the personality blooms."[137]

Jack La Lanne was also a proponent of the idea that exercise could supply energy and change one's personality. In his 1960 health guide, La Lanne, who regularly railed against the national epidemic of "pooped-out-itis," told readers that low energy levels were responsible for poor marital relations. "The wife who is weary after her day of housework doesn't come to the marriage-bed with the zest she did as a bride. How can she when she scarcely has the energy to drag through the day?"[138] La Lanne regularly addressed the segment of the television audience that, he was convinced, tuned in regularly but watched the show from the sofa. He divided his viewers into "sitters" and "doers." Using a poster board mounted on an easel, La Lanne displayed a visual rendering of these two types of viewers: doers were shown under a sunny sky, finding happiness through action and vitality; sitters were depicted looking sad, underneath a rain cloud.[139] During his show, La Lanne read letters from viewers who had lost weight or improved their physical condition. "Exercise can perform seeming miracles on our bodies and personalities," he wrote in a health guide for the over-forty set, helping to advance the notion that exercise was as valuable for minds as it was for bodies.[140]

The idea that exercise could provide extra energy or make for a happier disposition held wide appeal for women who failed to find fulfillment in housekeeping alone. The concept of exercise as cure-all proposed at least a partial solution to what Betty Friedan had labeled "the problem with no name."[141] Exercise could contribute to a thin and shapely figure and provide the energy to mother, attend to one's husband, keep house, and participate in civic activities, all the while helping to maintain a pleasant disposition. Exercise promoters made grand claims about the value of exercise, with their promises of physical transformation, energy acquisition, and personality improvement. These attributes had little if any relation to health, but they could help a woman better adjust to middle-class homemaking at midcentury. Throughout the 1960s, exercise functioned primarily as a beauty tool. As exercise discourse promoted the notion that the female body was purely decorative and that the value of exercise for

women lay in its ability to create a pleasing appearance, it reified traditional gender roles. At the same time, however, exercise discourse offered
women a regular opportunity to consider the care and functioning of their
bodies, an opportunity to engage in a leisure activity and take a moment
to think about themselves while family needs and household tasks took
second place.

Fitness culture of the 1960s encouraged the idea that the body was a
site of pleasure, but it also advocated self-surveillance. Figure control became part of the marriage bargain, but it also justified women devoting
time to themselves. As fitness entrepreneurs came to occupy an increasingly larger segment of popular culture, they worked to lengthen the list
of benefits exercise was said to bestow. Personal exuberance, dynamism,
and charisma were the result, they claimed, of a fully lived corporeal experience. While their promotional efforts indirectly upheld the notion that
a woman's place was in the home, they also unwittingly laid the foundation for women's participation in the jogging movement in the following
decade.

THE HEART OF THE MAN IN THE GRAY FLANNEL SUIT

MEN'S EXERCISE PROMOTION AND THE CARDIAC CRISIS

3

In 1962, an episode of the popular television series *Dennis the Menace* took on the subject of physical fitness. Dennis's neighbor, the curmudgeonly Mr. Wilson, receives a visit from his Uncle Ned, who, George Wilson tells young Dennis, has long been weak and feeble. When Uncle Ned arrives, however, he is the picture of health, delivering crushing handshakes and extolling the virtues of his new physical fitness regimen. Patting his pasty nephew's paunch, he chastises George and Dennis's father, Henry Mitchell, for their failure to exercise. "Don't you realize that our own president has said that we are a nation of underexercised push-button softies?" he asks, referring to John F. Kennedy. Both men's wives are in agreement with the latest statistics showing that American men don't get enough exercise as they age, and Alice Mitchell confides to Martha Wilson that she fears becoming a young widow. With the wives' support, Uncle Ned decides to share the joys of his fitness program with the reluctant Mitchell and Wilson, waking them at dawn for calisthenics and weight lifting. Ned's fitness tests prove that the two men are quite out of shape, but to silence their constant protests about the twice-daily workouts, Ned agrees to stop the training sessions if the two can match him in a weight-lifting contest. A comedic twist ensues when young Dennis easily lifts the supposedly heavy weights, revealing that Mitchell and Wilson have rigged the contest with a set of barbells made from lightweight balsa wood. Realizing that he has been had, Uncle Ned retaliates by scheduling the morning workout for an hour earlier.[1]

This humorous take on fitness encapsulates a number of new directions that exercise culture was taking in the 1960s. The episode links interest in exercise with federal exercise promotion efforts and President Kennedy, and it references the special emphasis on children's fitness—one of the reasons Henry Mitchell agrees to exercise is to set an example for young Dennis. The use of personal fitness as the central theme for an episode of a television show demonstrates Americans' growing awareness that exercise was an appropriate use of leisure time and that their bodies required such exercise for maintenance. But even as exercise grew in popularity, it continued to be, by and large, a chore performed out of obligation rather than a pleasurable activity, as evidenced by Henry and George's aversion to Ned's regimen. Finally, its depiction of spousal influence, and the fact that Martha and Alice encourage their husbands to exercise while refraining from doing so themselves, illustrates one of the central paradigms of exercise promotion in mid-twentieth-century America: for men, exercise was a question of health, a matter of life and death; for women, it was part of a beauty routine.

By the 1960s, in addition to popular exercise instructors and federal fitness efforts, scientific authorities had begun to weigh in about the benefits and risks of exercise. In medicine, the notion of preventive health care was growing. Research studies on diet, smoking, stress, and physical activity were revealing the influence of lifestyle on health.[2] Although many physicians had been persuaded that physical activity was an important component of longevity, there was no agreement on the value of exercise for health or weight loss. Some popular medical authorities, such as Paul Dudley White, urged Americans to get moving. Others, such as Peter Steincrohn, informed them that exercise was pointless and quite possibly dangerous. And even if doctors could agree that exercising was advisable, exactly what counted as exercise and the optimal length of time one should do so remained unclear. In the absence of consensus, popular and expert authorities, who were growing in both number and influence, spoke out loudly for and against exercise and, in the process, made it difficult for

Americans to discern whether and how they should integrate it into their lives.

When Alice Mitchell related her fear of widowhood to Martha Wilson, the audience clearly understood that she was worried that Henry might have a heart attack. Beginning in the early 1950s, the "menace that strikes without warning" took on epidemic proportions and escalated into a nationwide panic about the state of men's health that lasted through the 1960s.[3] As the media described it, American men were dying in unprecedented numbers, felled by a silent and unpredictable killer that struck them in the prime of their lives. Tales of men's sudden demise during their commute, at their desks, and on the golf course formed the basis for magazine articles and novels; such stories were recounted in excruciating detail in survival narratives and provided fodder for at least one motion picture parody.[4] When President Dwight Eisenhower, whose trim figure bespoke his military training and well-known golf habit, suffered a heart attack in 1955, it seemed as if anyone could be struck anytime, anywhere. The nationwide panic about the state of men's hearts prompted a surge in the publication of health guides for men. This body of literature played a crucial role in widening the discussion about exercise to include medical and scientific experts and, in the process, legitimated exercise as a leisure pursuit.

Before the 1960s, popular exercise promoters who targeted an adult clientele were largely self-taught, and the profession's reputation was somewhat spurious. Physical educators with college degrees typically worked in educational institutions, leaving adult-oriented fitness instruction in the hands of well-meaning amateurs and less well-meaning hucksters. Writing in 1966, cardiologist Carleton Chapman noted that, until recently, "physical vigor was not a concern of the American adult, the topic was more or less suspect; the compulsive focus of health faddists rather than the legitimate interest of the rank and file."[5] A new focus on preventive health care in the 1960s meant that many physicians began to provide health advice and speak out on lifestyle choices. For men, this led to the development of a new genre of consumer health manuals that targeted "executive health"—an emerging specialty devoted to the specific needs of middle- and upper-class white men who worked at high-pressure desk jobs and lived a primarily suburban existence. The combination of executive health guides and heart attack prevention literature (whose target audiences were nearly identical) brought national attention to men's health and to exercise for health's sake. Authored primarily by physicians, whose prestige lent credibility to these publications, men's health literature encouraged physical activity yet created uncertainty at the same time. "Exercise" remained a vague and undefined notion through most of the decade; moreover, for middle-class men, it held little cultural appeal, either as a display of virtue or as an appearance enhancer.

THE CARDIAC CRISIS

Physicians had been observing a rise in the rate of heart attacks since the 1920s.[6] At midcentury, this increase appeared particularly dramatic because it was coupled with a number of advancements in public health that had decreased the incidence of other illnesses and created the perception of a new and fast-growing problem. The development of antibiotics and major progress against diseases related to sanitation and infection had eliminated many of the nation's top causes of death by the late 1950s. In the decade between 1944 and 1954, for example, death rates had fallen precipitously from diseases such as influenza (91 percent decline), appendicitis (76 percent), rheumatic fever (73 percent), tuberculosis (73 percent), and syphilis (63 percent).[7] These advances increased longevity in the population as a whole, which meant that late-in-life chronic diseases became more common. In addition, diagnostic methods and disease categorization had become more sophisticated and systematized in the late 1940s and early 1950s, resulting in a more precise measurement of the number of deaths attributable to coronary heart disease, in which blood flow in the arteries leading to the heart is limited or blocked altogether.[8] By 1956, coronary heart disease was identified as the leading cause of death in men aged thirty and older.[9] Even more troubling was evidence that coronary heart disease was being found in increasingly younger men. Autopsies on American soldiers killed in the Korean War revealed that men in their twenties and thirties were showing signs of atherosclerosis, a buildup of plaque in the arteries that is a precursor of coronary heart disease.[10]

At the same time, it was becoming clear to physicians that not all men were at equal risk. Medical and epidemiological studies conducted through the midcentury period had established that lifestyle factors played a significant role in one's propensity for having a heart attack. Nutrition researcher Ancel Keys's work during the 1950s on the relationship among cholesterol, fat, and disease, as well as his comparison of disease rates and diet in several countries, helped identify diet as a source of risk.[11] In Britain, studies by Heady and Morris noted differences in the health and bodies of men whose jobs required physical activity. Their work comparing the health of London bus drivers, who were sedentary, with the health of ticket takers, who walked the aisles of double-decker buses throughout the day, was a crucial first step in correlating exercise and good health.[12] Finally, stress was also examined for its role in causing heart attacks. Walter Cannon's theory of the "fight or flight syndrome," developed in 1915 but popular in the 1950s, held that without physical release, men (especially "desk-bound" executives) were unable to slough off the day's stress through activity, and thus their bodies were subjected to the corrosive effects of stress hormones.[13] The sum of these and other studies gradually established the notion that health was the result not of luck but of lifestyle, giving media-savvy physicians a new importance in popular culture.

The escalation of heart disease in men occurred at a particularly vulnerable time in American history, when gender roles were in flux and cultural critics feared that the American male was in decline. The emphasis on the nuclear family and "togetherness," women's growing power in the home and workplace, and corporations' need for workers who could submit to hierarchy unsettled long-established patterns of life in the United States. Men of the postwar era felt that their cultural dominance was being challenged and sensed a loss of individuality and independence.[14] In 1958, the editors of Look magazine summed up these feelings in an illustrated book titled The Decline of the American Male, which only half-humorously asked "Why Do Women Dominate Him?" "Why Is He Afraid to Be Different?" and "Why Does He Work so Hard?"[15] The rising rate of heart attacks in men seemed to offer proof that the cultural shifts reflected in these chapter titles were untenable.

Barbara Ehrenreich was the first historian to recognize the cultural significance of the midcentury cardiac crisis. Using a feminist framework to evaluate the panic, she argued that the heart attack epidemic, especially

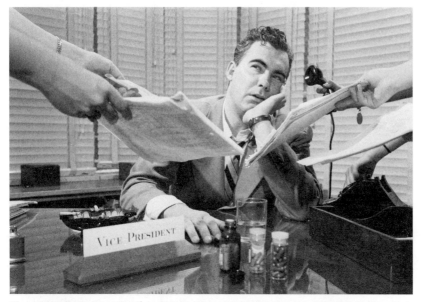

Throughout the 1950s and 1960s, the state of men's mental and physical health was a national preoccupation. "Desk-bound" jobs, the stress of white-collar employment, and a dramatic increase in heart attacks encouraged the belief that men's bodies required special care. (© Phillip A. Harrington, photographer, Look Magazine Photograph Collection, Prints and Photographs Division, Library of Congress, LC Job 52-1238-Frame 1)

its linkages to white-collar employment and stress, was actually part of a pattern of male rebellion against the breadwinner role. Men could invoke overstress and overwork to exempt themselves from the demands of career and family. Financially dependent wives would have to learn to live within their means or risk losing their husbands to heart attacks.[16] Ehrenreich's analysis focused almost exclusively on stress, which was a relatively new concept—even the term was new, popularized by researcher Hans Selye in a 1956 book—but it overlooked larger cultural and physical changes occurring as a result of new work patterns, new eating trends, and new modes of living.[17]

The suburban commuter lifestyle, heavy smoking, the three-martini business lunch, and long hours made for an unhealthy and stressful life-style. One study of Chicago businessmen showed that the average chief executive worked a fifty-three-hour week and brought another ten hours of work home.[18] In families with only one wage earner, the pressure to perform and provide was substantial. The Decline of the American Male pointed out that the consumption of tranquilizers, barbiturates, and alcohol was growing, along with the sale of "how-to-relax books."[19] A psychiatrist working with white-collar businessmen affirmed that "stress and executive anxiety are endemic. Desks are full of pills. Liquor for lunch is a necessity."[20]

Experts seemed to agree that middle-class men with desk jobs were prone to exceptional stresses. In 1957, for example, the topic of the American Management Association's annual meeting was "The Man in Management," directly and indirectly addressing charges of conformity made in William Whyte's The Organization Man. Papers presented at the conference highlighted how men as individuals were important to business, with a special focus on health and "tension relieving."[21] In the 1950s and 1960s, the American College of Physicians similarly featured panels on "the care and protection of the American executive" at annual meetings.[22] The emergence of "executive health" as a medical subspecialty furthered the belief that the health of executives, and particularly their hearts, required special handling. Originating from the field of occupational medicine, executive health had been developing since the 1940s—a time when employees often spent their entire careers with one firm—as large companies with medical directors began to offer physical examinations and medical testing to ensure productivity and reduce absenteeism.[23]

A portrait of the stereotypical heart attack victim emerged during this time (and continues to dominate the popular imagination): He was a white, middle-aged, hardworking husband and father employed as a mid-level manager or executive. He was a suburban dweller who endured a long commute into the city. He smoked to relieve stress, drank too much, and had no time for physical activity other than weekend golf. He made little time for vacations or personal hobbies and put his own interests behind the needs and desires of his family. The author of Managing Your Coronary described the typical victim as a man over the age of forty-five, "a busy office worker or executive, always hurried, always overworked . . . an ambitious individual—you drive yourself hard . . . an unhappy man at home, your wife seems to be always complaining and your children are quarrelsome and impertinent."[24]

The belief that men's hearts were in danger was a critique of consumption, a prolongation of the discussion of the effects of affluence and ambition that had characterized the postwar era. That so many men were succumbing to a sudden, often fatal, illness just as the nation was finally enjoying a measure of political stability and economic prosperity seemed a cruel twist of fate. As the authors of one consumer health guide expressed it, employing a phrase that referred to both postwar affluence and the new suburban lifestyle: "Heart disease has risen to tragic prominence at a time when so many Americans are enjoying the 'good life' and prosperity. The horrid thought is inescapable that somehow this epidemic is fundamentally due to aspects of our new modern way of life."[25]

As the earlier excerpt from *Managing Your Coronary* illustrates, the cultural construction of the unhappy husband burdened by family life certainly did exist. Ehrenreich's analysis pointed out that men were thought to be at risk because their wives desired material goods. In 1954, for example, *Cosmopolitan* ran an epistolary confessional entitled "I'm to Blame that My Husband Died Too Young," in which Jane Lincoln explains to her sister that her desire for a fur coat, a television, a dress for her daughter, and a new bike for her son caused her husband's fatal heart attack.[26] But just as often, men were depicted as eager to climb the corporate ladder; not striving for career advancement was considered unmanly. As the female author of a 1956 *Saturday Evening Post* article put it, "Men are always going to think it is sissy to ease up, unless we want to change their minds."[27]

While the *Cosmopolitan* article made it plain that wives needed to control their material longings, it also highlighted men's role in the acquisition of goods, the need to keep up and get ahead in business. Alongside the story, the magazine ran a photo-essay featuring businessman Rudolph Sittler reacting to the article and the ideas within it. Sittler recognized himself and his family in the narrative as "headed for needless tragedy," and he asked, "Just where did I think I was going?" Sittler's choice of pronoun, as well as the accompanying photos, illustrated that men were complicit in the new postwar economy of affluence, but as the magazine pointed out, the problem was "how to slow the merry-go-round without getting off."[28] Rather than perceiving the cardiac crisis as men's attempt to flee commitment, it might be more helpful to see it as part of the adjustment process as Americans learned to adapt to a new environment that no longer took the body into consideration—a first stab at achieving what we now call work-life balance.

While no wife wanted her husband to suffer a heart attack, surviving one was almost a badge of honor—victims earned membership in the Pump Club, the Coronary Club, or the Royal Coronia Society. But it wasn't the triumph of health over disease that warranted admiration—it was a perverse sense of pride at being afflicted in the first place. Some observers theorized that the desirable characteristics that made a man successful in business were the same ones that put his health at risk. As the medical director of one large corporation asserted, "The intrinsic qualities which make men able executives, such as imagination and driving energy, are the very ones which may lead to disaster."[29] In his guide to executive health, physician Charles Thompson surmised that if his readers were executives, they must "be in possession of above-average intelligence, above-average ambitions, above-average ability and above-average self-discipline."[30] Although knowledge about the risks of high cholesterol, cigarette smoking, and a sedentary lifestyle was rapidly expanding, the attribution of moralistic qualities to heart attacks helped blunt the effects of suffering one. In 1954, physician W. Melville Arnott suggested that "the 'stress and strain' theory" was popular because "it nourishes the [self-esteem] of the believer and it is readily acceptable to the unfortunate victim and his relatives. It places ischemic heart disease in the position of being the unjust reward of virtue. How much nicer it is when stricken with a coronary thrombosis to be told it is all due to hard work, laudable ambition and a selfless devotion to duty."[31] Consider the profile developed by physiologist Irvine Page of the man who was *not* coronary prone:

He is an effeminate municipal worker or embalmer, completely lacking in physical and mental alertness, without drive, ambition, or competitive spirit, who has never attempted to meet a deadline at any time. He is a man with poor appetite, subsisting on fruits and vegetables, laced with corn and whale oil, detesting tobacco, and spurning ownership of a TV, radio, or motor car. He has a full head of hair, and is scrawny and unathletic in appearance, yet he is constantly straining his puny muscles by exercise. He is low in income, blood pressure, blood sugar, uric acid, and cholesterol. He has been on nicotinic acid, pyridoxine, and anti-coagulant therapy ever since his prophylactic castration.[32]

This reverse characterization rejects victimization and suggests that some men claimed their susceptibility to heart disease with a morbid glee, the weakness of their hearts demonstrating their masculinity. Given that, during this era, middle-class men's worth was demonstrated primarily by their ability to support their families, it is logical that some men resented the notion that their wives were demanding too much and instead took pride in their business acumen and ability to provide.

One result of the construct of executive heart attack victim, however, was the erroneous and widespread belief that men outside this class were not at risk. (Women's risk of heart disease was rarely discussed, as they were believed to be immune until after menopause.) Working-class men were largely thought to be exempt from heart disease because of the physical nature of their work. The notion that white-collar work is somehow singularly unhealthy has a long history. Sociologist William Rothstein documented numerous sources from the 1920s, 1930s, and 1940s that correlated the prevalence of heart attacks with class position.[33] In the 1950s and 1960s, media coverage of the cardiac crisis continued to perpetuate the association between heart attacks and middle- and upper-class status.[34] Despite a long chronology of studies that disproved this theory, the links among white-collar office work, class, and heart disease remained stubbornly in place at midcentury.[35]

It is likely that these beliefs about heart disease had cultural antecedents in the turn-of-the-century neurasthenia "epidemic." In the nineteenth century, neurologist George Beard promoted the idea that the strain of "brain work" could cause sickness. In his 1881 book *American Nervousness*, Beard described neurasthenia, a vague and ill-defined malady with diverse symptoms that included dyspepsia, depression, sweaty hands, and yawning. Neurasthenia emerged as an illness just as corporations began to dominate the American economy, creating a need for new kinds of workers. Between the 1880s and 1920s—a period that resembled the mid-twentieth century in terms of workplace transformation—salesmen, managers, and other midlevel executives expanded in number and kind in a new, hierarchical labor force that seemingly had no use for entrepreneurship and individualism, values that had previously given men's work meaning. A catch-all term and cultural construct, neurasthenia was less a disease than a reflection of men's uneasiness with the new nonproductive culture of labor. Neurasthenia as a diagnosis gradually fell out of favor in the early twentieth century, but the idea that white-collar men were prone to special kinds of illnesses did not. The notion that "brain work" without the release of physical labor could make a man ill was buoyed by the 1950s cardiac crisis. Whereas men from that earlier era could reinvigorate their health through physical pursuits, which were tremendously popular at the time, this option was not readily available to midcentury men. Moreover, just as a heart attack could function as evidence of a businessman's ambition and drive, neurasthenia symbolized a certain level of superiority, although in the earlier period, it was marked more by racial than class overtones. As historian Harvey Green has pointed out, "primitive" groups, including workers of color and marginalized social groups, were immune to neurasthenia. The disease afflicted primarily members of "civilized" society.[36]

Although class issues were evident in the perception of heart attack risk, it seems that race did not function in the same way. Heart attacks apparently did not afflict the African American community to the same degree as the white population. Mortality rates from coronary heart disease were found to be significantly higher among white men in statistical surveys compiled by the Metropolitan Life Insurance Company and for *Vital Statistics of the United States*, although African Americans had higher mortality rates in all other disease categories. William Rothstein's statistical analysis of early-twentieth-century mortality rates concludes that "coronary heart disease was predominantly a disease of white rather than black men." Rothstein persuasively refutes the possibility that diagnostic bias (resulting from the coronary-prone profile) played a role in the findings.[37] A separate 1957 study involving more than 15,000 subjects in St. Louis, Washington, D.C., and New Orleans similarly found that black Americans had one-fifth the rate of coronary thrombosis of white Americans.[38] African American newspapers such as the *Chicago Defender* and the *Baltimore Afro-American* covered cardiac health (primarily wire reports), but they did not succumb to the panicked reporting of other publications of the era, another indication that heart attacks were not perceived as a significant threat to black men's health.

The racial discrepancy in heart disease was likely because African Americans did not yet enjoy the affluent lifestyle that led to increased rates of heart disease among white Americans. One 1966 study that compared rates of atherosclerosis in black Americans and in Haitians also supported environmental factors, including diet, stress, and physical conditioning, as causative. Dale Groom, the lead author of the study, noted that "human muscles do daily [in Haiti] what has since been relegated to machines in our civilization," echoing previous laments about the changing nature of the physical environment. The *Baltimore Afro-American* similarly placed blame on lifestyle, noting that "this study is a measure of what our American way of life does to a race with regard to coronary heart disease."[39] As part of the working class, most black men were assumed to obtain sufficient exercise to ward off heart disease. Consequently, heart attack prevention literature and executive health manuals focused exclusively on white men.

MEN'S HEALTH ADVICE

The primacy of the nuclear family in the postwar era and men's role as breadwinner meant that men's heart disease affected the entire family. When a man died of a heart attack, it was a terrible loss, but depictions of the consequences focused as much on the loss of the man as on the future suffering of his impoverished family, his lonely wife, and his fatherless children. The United States had become, in the words of one *Saturday Evening Post* writer, "a country awash with widows."[40] This view helps explain why a large portion of heart attack prevention literature was written not for men but for their wives. During the 1950s and 1960s, magazines, manufacturers, physicians, and even the American Heart Association targeted the female audience to encourage men to adopt heart-healthy behaviors, while male-oriented business and style magazines remained largely silent on the topic. To protect their husbands, wives were supposed to set good examples, reduce stress in the home, serve nutritious meals, make smart buying decisions, and even resort to subterfuge when resistant husbands balked at their efforts. On the one hand, such positioning relegated women to the traditional role of nursemaid, but on the other hand, it increased women's power within the household. The same heart attack narratives that advised women to curb their material desires also recommended that they step up and take charge of their husbands, their homes, and their families. Decisions related to meal planning, home management, and purchasing were cloaked in an aura of scientific expertise that the wife alone had mastered, allowing her to make decisions for the family from a position of heightened authority. Unfortunately, such delegation also encouraged men to abdicate responsibility for their own health.

Dietary advice was the most logical arena to encourage women's interest in heart attack prevention, given that wives were responsible for meal preparation in most middle-class homes. Growing knowledge of cholesterol's role in heart disease made a heart-healthy diet "the first line of defense against the nation's number one killer."[41] Prevention-oriented cookbooks constituted a new and popular culinary subgenre in the 1950s and 1960s, with some, such as Ancel and Margaret Keys's *Eat Well and Stay Well*, becoming best sellers.[42] Women's magazines also devoted considerable attention to heart attack prevention in their food pages. Although men were the potential victims, their wives were supposed to learn the difference between saturated and unsaturated fat and which foods contained high levels of cholesterol. They could then plan meals accordingly, and their husbands were sometimes unaware that they had been put on diets. In *Reader's Digest*, for example, cardiologist Herman Sobol recommended that "rather than have scenes at the table about his eating the fat on the roast, remove the fat in the kitchen."[43]

Women were encouraged to extend their efforts beyond the kitchen to include nearly all aspects of men's preventive health care. Wives, according to prominent cardiologist Jeremiah Stamler, were the "guardian of family health." His consumer guide, *Your Heart Has Nine Lives*, encouraged women to become experts on the topic of heart disease. "Look at your husband," the book pleaded: "Is he the slim young man he was five to ten or twenty or thirty years ago? Are you giving him more food than he really needs, or the wrong kinds? . . . Are his arteries healthy, or rusting, or is he—and can you know? . . . Or is he drifting like millions of others closer to disaster? From knowledge about this artery disease, a wife can help her husband reduce his risks."[44]

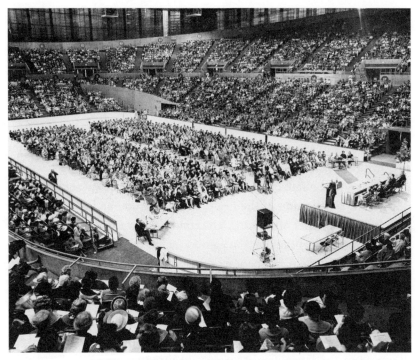

More than 10,000 women attended "Hearts and Husbands," a conference sponsored by the Oregon Heart Association to teach caring wives how to help their husbands avoid heart disease. As the "guardians of family health," wives were expected to become familiar with the signs of a heart attack, prepare special diets, and reduce stress in the home. (The Harvard Medical Library in the Francis A. Countway Library of Medicine)

According to the physician-author of the 1962 book *How Not to Kill Your Husband*, it was not normal for a man to "fuss about his health." Kenneth C. Hutchin confided to readers, "Although they would never admit it, even the most difficult husbands regard it as a wife's responsibility to look after their health. If they don't, no one else will—until too late."[45] Boston cardiologist Paul Dudley White similarly advised wives to lighten family meals and to persuade their husbands to stop smoking and to exercise.[46] White was an avid proponent of regular exercise for health and was known to take frequent bicycle rides near his home in Massachusetts. He had gained a national reputation when he cared for Eisenhower after the president's heart attack; White's prescription for exercise flew in the face

of traditional recovery plans that called for the patient's near immobiliza-
tion for weeks after the incident and a long recovery at home.[47]

In 1964, White was invited to give the keynote speech at "Hearts and
Husbands," a women-only health conference sponsored by the Oregon
Heart Association. The free event was widely promoted and was scheduled
at lunchtime so that wives could be home in time to serve dinner. Charter
buses from around the state brought the female attendees, who filled Memorial Coliseum's 10,000 seats, and created an unprecedented traffic jam
in downtown Portland. Besides White's remarks to "Wives and sisters,
mothers and daughters," there were exhibits of cardiology equipment, a
film on the functioning of the heart, and a question-and-answer period
with White and other physicians. The conference was considered so successful that it was repeated in San Francisco, Salt Lake City (at the Mormon
Tabernacle, with the participation of the choir), and elsewhere in reduced
form through the 1960s.[48]

Televised public-service announcements for the American Heart Association's annual door-to-door fund-raising drive also drove home the
notion that women were responsible for their families' health. A spot
produced in the late 1960s, "A Salute to the American Wife," stressed
the importance of women's involvement in family health while appearing to mock the drudgery of homemaking. A montage of still photos of
unhappy wives doing chores was paired with a semihumorous narration
that upgraded housekeeping tasks to important-sounding responsibilities
(ironing became "home maintenance," cooking was "food management,"
mending required a "reconstruction expert," and chauffeuring children
necessitated a "transportation expediter"). Presumably, however, the spot
did not intend to imply that women's role as health guardian was a joke.
As footage showed an extended family returning home from an outing,
the narrator encouraged mothers and wives to give to the Heart Fund volunteer (always female) as he boomed, "That's why the American wife has
made heart her cause. . . . She's the guardian of her family's health."[49]

Wives' efforts were considered equally essential when it came to stress
reduction. While they could do little to alter their husbands' work environments, they could create a stress-free zone inside the home for the health
and comfort of their husbands.[50] Women were urged to control the chil-

dren when Dad arrived home from work, allowing him to have a cocktail and unwind. "If you can introduce an element of restfulness at homecoming time, you're making a real contribution," one physician advised.[51] Ehrenreich's theory that the cardiac crisis was a form of rebellion rings true with regard to stress. Husbands could exempt themselves from undesirable chores, citing the risk of a heart attack. In his consumer health guide *If Your Husband Has Coronary Heart Disease*, cardiologist Robert Sonneborn noted some of these advantages "to the husband with heart disease. He has a built-in excuse. In fact he may get away with things which make healthy males envious. . . . No more grass cutting when there is a good program on TV. Cleaning the attic or garage is taboo. Someone else carries the luggage, and you are no longer a lush—a drink is just what the doctor ordered. Poor Dad!"[52]

Not surprisingly, several 1960s advertising campaigns used the cardiac crisis to promote products that reified women's position as their husbands' health guardians while also emphasizing the gravity of their purchasing choices. In text-heavy, somber advertisements, companies such as Mazola (margarine and cooking oil), D-Zerta (gelatin), Metropolitan Life (insurance), Beautyrest (mattresses), and Jockey (underwear) all explained how their products could contribute to male health while "informing" readers of *Ladies' Home Journal* and *Good Housekeeping* about men's health issues. Mazola educated readers on the dangers of saturated fat. Metropolitan Life suggested that couples make joint appointments for physicals: "Many wives have learned the simple trick of saying '*we* should have a physical examination' and going with their husbands to the doctor's."[53] Beautyrest asked, "Is one-third of his life worth anything to you?" and likened a poor night's sleep to "man-killing fatigue," explaining how a reduced heart rate at night could potentially save a hardworking (male) heart thousands of beats.[54] Jockey made the question "boxers or briefs?" a health issue when the company argued that its patented undergarment designed by a urological surgeon could prevent male "self-injury."[55] The existence of these campaigns speaks to how extensively the male health crisis permeated popular culture, while the placement of these ads exclusively in women's magazines demonstrates the degree to which men were absolved from caring for their own health.

EXERCISE FOR MEN

One advantage of the commercial nature of women's exercise promotion was that there were a number of sources of information, allowing women to decide for themselves whether a particular instructor, book, or record was worthwhile. This contrasted greatly with men's exercise promotion in the 1960s, which, though spurred by health concerns, offered far fewer courses of action. Exercise was promoted as one piece of a multipronged approach to preventing heart disease. But rarely did this information offer specifics akin to the diet plans and exercise instructions outlined in women's magazines. This patchwork approach to health promotion meant that many consumers were in the dark about the type, duration, and intensity of activity suitable for at-risk men. And truth be told, many men had no interest in exercise. As the previously described *Dennis the Menace* episode made clear, exercise held little appeal for the George Wilsons and Henry Mitchells of the world.

With their bodies hidden under suit jackets, most middle-class men simply didn't give much thought to body maintenance for the sake of aesthetics.[56] Grooming and charm were considered more important qualities than bulging biceps or even broad shoulders. This is not to say that issues such as hair loss and a trim waist were unimportant to middle-class men; however, the qualities that typically motivate contemporary American men to exercise, such as musculature and corpulence, and their attendant social pressures, were largely absent from men's advice literature.

Magazines aimed at a white middle-class readership, such as *Esquire*, *Gentlemen's Quarterly*, and *Playboy*, rarely covered diet or exercise issues, despite significant attention to men's fashion and grooming products. Even when these publications did discuss overweight, it was presented not as a personal failure, a barrier to finding a mate, or a health issue but as an obstacle to dressing in the latest fashions. Writer Tom Burke's *GQ* articles about his own weight loss described his motivation as stemming from a desire to wear up-to-date clothing, not to achieve a perfect physique. "I secretly admired the trend to slim-cut clothes," he admitted, "but I went right on wearing wide cuffs and jackets bought before the last World's Fair. . . . Where the clothes tapered I did not. . . . I looked like a malformed eggplant."[57] Historian Lynne Luciano notes that even the men pictured in *Playboy* were "well-dressed, usually fully clothed, looking less sensual than successful, less vain about their bodies than their clothing and cars."[58] Todd Olszewski notes a similar absence of concern for the body's exterior in his study of heart-healthy diet plans of the 1950s and 1960s. Although men who followed diets to reduce cholesterol and prevent heart attacks likely lost weight, low-fat diets were valued primarily for the "physiological, rather than the physical," changes they effected.[59] Dieting to achieve a better figure was largely understood as a feminine undertaking.[60] The absence of attention to the male body is curious, given the significant coverage devoted to what GQ called in 1964 "the new sport of consummate grooming."[61] The magazine noted that over the previous ten years, the range of men's consumer products had expanded exponentially to include items such as cologne, face masks, blemish concealers, and hair-care products, all of which, it should be noted, were designed for use above the shoulders.[62]

It is highly likely that the reason men distanced themselves from their bodies was that the act of observing and inspecting one's physique and those of other men was tinged by the specter of homosexuality. Dominique Padurano has persuasively argued that Charles Atlas and his mail-order bodybuilding course helped refashion gender roles for working-class and ethnic men in the first half of the century, allowing for self-comparison and the inspection of other men's bodies. Atlas's popularization of bodybuilding "helped to make homoaestheticism a requisite component of twentieth-century heteronormative masculinity."[63] For middle-class men, however, this shift did not occur until the late 1970s with the expansion of the fitness club industry, a new class of film stars, and the rise of the singles scene. As a result, negative associations among homosexuality, diminished intelligence, and attention to the body worked to disconnect middle-class men from their physical selves for much of the century.

The muscular male body in pictorial magazines of the 1950s and 1960s—whether shown to promote fitness culture or for titillation purposes—supported the notion that "upstanding" men paid little attention to their appearance. Being too preoccupied with the development of one's physique could invite speculation about one's sexuality. Bodybuilding magazines, such as those published by fitness impresario Joe Weider, were virtually indistinguishable from Bob Mizer's *Physique Pictorial*, which served a primarily gay readership. F. Valentine Hooven argues that the muscle magazines of the 1950s and 1960s were, in fact, "the first 'gay' magazines." The boundaries between the two types of publications were porous: images of Hollywood actors could often be found in both, and heterosexual bodybuilders in need of income often posed for gay-oriented magazines. Once Weider realized the scope of the gay market, he knowingly expanded his offerings to attract gay readers.[64] *Playboy* made the association between muscles and sexuality clear in a 1967 cartoon depicting two bodybuilders attempting to woo a woman on a beach; then they take notice of each other's bodies, abandon their attempts to seduce the woman, and go off together instead.[65]

In addition to spawning fears of homosexuality, an overly muscular physique created the perception of diminished intelligence in the minds of many Americans. Even Jack La Lanne, who clearly displayed his physique in a form-fitting jumpsuit on his television show, risked being thought of as dumb. La Lanne's business manager confided to one interviewer, "Of course, we try to play down Jack's muscles. I don't mean there's anything wrong with having muscles, it's just that people tend to associate a muscular body with a muscle-bound mind."[66] In the same vein, *Esquire* produced a three-page spread poking fun at John F. Kennedy's high-profile efforts to promote fitness for Americans in 1962. The magazine depicted Kennedy as a hugely muscular caveman in a leopard-print brief, in a parody of Charles Atlas's well-known ninety-eight-pound weakling ads.[67]

A regular exercise habit for its own sake had few positive moralistic associations for middle-class men. Whereas notions of virtue, self-control, and discipline were an integral part of the appeal of the Atlas bodybuilding course for working-class men, these attributes were demonstrated in other ways for middle-class men—notably, by their abilities as wage earners, family providers, and fathers.[68] It would be a few more years before the jogging movement and the creation of workplace fitness centers aligned the concepts of professional capability and physical prowess. Of the few advertisements in middle-class men's magazines that referenced appearance or body shape, the majority were for devices relying on electrical stimulation to improve muscle tone. One advertisement for the Relax-a-Cizor, for example, depicted a thoughtful-looking man with the device's belt wrapped around his waist, while he held a book in one hand and a drink and a cigarette in the other, clearly illustrating that there was no virtue in physical activity.[69]

When exercise for men was discussed, it was often valued more for its tension-relieving qualities than its ability to develop muscles or tone the body. The back cover of Bonnie Prudden's exercise record *Executive Fitness*, for example, explained the fight-or-flight response in the context of work and described the residual physical effects on the male body after a stressful moment at the office: "That magnificent fighting machine . . . just has to sit there with all engines howling . . . and take it . . . often with a smile. When it's all over he feels as though he had shaken himself to pieces. . . . His neck and shoulders hurt, he develops ulcers, his vitality and virility ebb . . . and finally there's a pain in his heart." To release stress, Prudden recommended ten minutes of exercise from her program of light calisthenics, stretching, and running in place.[70] Prudden was one of the few who offered a specific course of action that men could take to improve their health. Her depiction of a masterful, powerful man who has to subsume his forceful, natural impulses for the sake of corporate hierarchy exemplified midcentury thinking that American business culture was harmful to men's health.

Over the course of the 1960s, as more studies revealed a link between a decreased risk of heart attack and increased physical activity, exercise for the sake of activity was recommended for men. But details on the optimal intensity, duration, and frequency of exercise were often so vague or subject to such variation that men may have had difficulty determining which advice was credible. Executive health guides and popular articles on heart attack prevention repeatedly stated the need for some kind of exercise but rarely addressed the specifics. Typical of the media coverage was an interview in *Nation's Business* with E. Garland Herndon, a physician who specialized in executive health. When asked what exercises "a desk-bound businessman" should follow, Herndon responded, "Exercise should vary from executive to executive depending on what is available to him, what his interests are and the time that he has to accomplish them," leaving the reader to guess at what approach to take.[71] Most books typically devoted just a few pages to physical activity, spending more time discussing whether to take up exercise than what activities to do. In his executive health guide, for instance, physician Charles Thompson emphasized the importance of regular exercise to improve health and reduce stress, but he had relatively few practical suggestions.[72] Physician Harry Johnson recognized that most men would have difficulty incorporating exercise into their daily routines, given their already tight schedules. He recommended getting an hour of exercise a day, which included stretching in bed after the alarm rang, using one's towel "vigorously," bending over "all the way" to pick up one's socks, and performing isometric buttocks contractions while waiting for the elevator. Although Johnson's suggestions demonstrate an awareness of the need for physical activity, they also illustrate how ill equipped physicians were to design exercise programs for their patients, and they attest to the sedate nature of midcentury exercise.[73]

One reason that so little exercise information was provided to men was the assumption that most had received adequate physical training as boys in school sports programs or as young men in the military and could rely on that background to design their own exercise programs. Experts often warned, however, that if performed incorrectly, physical activity could be dangerous or even fatal. Exercise physiologist Thomas Cureton advised men not to engage in the sports of their youth, such as basketball and handball, because these were "high-tension" activities—that is, they were competitive and involved short bursts of high energy, which, he believed, could endanger the heart and result in blood vessel damage.[74] Dr. A. L. Chapman, assistant surgeon general of the United States, similarly warned that exercise could be dangerous: "if [an individual] hasn't been taking exercise in a long time, he can assume that he's out of condition—that any sudden excessive exercise may kill him."[75] Participating in competitive sports also required caution, because the stress-relieving benefits were likely to be outweighed by men's competitive urges. "Under the duress of excitement and drive to win, the heart patient may not be willing to stop when he feels the danger signals," *Sports Illustrated* warned.[76] Moreover, men were instructed not to force themselves to do something they didn't enjoy, because the resulting stress would negate any benefits the exercise bestowed; thus, beneficial but dull activities, such as calisthenics, were also ill-advised.[77]

When it came to specific activities, walking, hiking, bowling, golfing, swimming, and occasionally tennis were typically suggested for men.[78] But activities that required a partner or took a long time (such as playing eighteen holes of golf) were difficult to manage during the workweek, and experts also advised against becoming a weekend athlete.[79] Fearful of excessive exertion and unable to rely on the sports backgrounds they had developed in their youth, middle-aged men were ill equipped to begin exercising on their own.

Adding to the plethora of confusing health information was a stream of contradictory advice that any kind of exercise program could be dangerous. Although millions of Americans were beginning to accept the notion that physical activity was a necessary adjustment to modern life, there were opponents who argued that exercise was a needless waste of energy and that it could even be deadly. In his syndicated newspaper column and numerous books, cardiologist Peter Steincrohn warned of the dangers of "exercisitis," a malady that could be spread by a single doctor to "a few thousand laymen. Multiply such proponents of physical fitness by the many who follow in sheeplike credulity, and you have the reason for the present epidemic of physical contortions sweeping the United States."[80] His book How to Be Lazy, Healthy and Fit, which featured chapters such as "Rest Begins at 40" and "Americans Are Too Exercise-Conscious," argued that exercise was unnecessary for good health. It wasn't that Steincrohn didn't believe in exercise at all; rather, he disagreed with the growing sentiment, demonstrated by La Lanne and other fitness enthusiasts, that exercise was a panacea for all illness. Even more fervently, Steincrohn resisted the notion of exercise as a fountain of youth. One of the goals of his book was to counter a spate of works that informed readers how to get more out of life in middle age and beyond.[81]

Steincrohn was fully aware of the numerous studies suggesting that exercise cleared cholesterol from the body and led to better health. He disagreed with such research based on its methodology and on the wisdom he had accumulated over twenty-five years of practicing medicine. Instead, he argued that an individual was born with a finite number of heartbeats and that exercise consumed too many of these; as a result, heart attacks often followed vigorous exercise. "Cease or decease!" he grimly warned.[82]

Steincrohn was a firm believer in rest and relaxation and the notion that men and women should do nothing whenever possible. His opinions were grounded in an appreciation of the trappings of modern life. He disagreed with those who lamented the passing of a more physical past. "The good old days? Who wants them?" he asked, comparing the ease of using the starter button on his car with the annoyance of cranking a Model T.[83] Steincrohn's resistance to the burgeoning fitness movement was, no doubt, shared by many. Reviews of his book in small local newspapers indicated that not all Americans were ready to embrace exercise. "His books are comfort indeed to those of us who feel guilty about physical laziness," the *Anniston (Alabama) Star* commiserated.[84]

Steincrohn's book was published in 1968, near the end of a decade that saw popular opinion about the value of exercise shift dramatically. Even if they didn't partake of the new trend, Americans were gradually becoming convinced of the need to exercise, thanks to medical news, popular culture, and sporting goods manufacturers. But teaching Americans to enjoy exercise was another matter entirely. TV exercise personality Debbie Drake reportedly gave up on her career after finding that she couldn't motivate clients beyond an initial period of three or four months.[85] One of Steincrohn's main objections to exercise was that men and women would be incapable of keeping up a regular activity that relied on willpower and discipline, rather than pleasure, to motivate them. "Not only do [most people] not think exercise is fun, they actually hate it," he attested.[86]

While numerous authorities took advantage of a profitable environment to tell women how to exercise, few targeted the male population. Thomas Cureton, who ran the Physical Fitness Laboratory at the University of Illinois, was one of the few experts for men, but because he worked mainly in academic circles and with professional associations, his popular influence was limited. Cureton's vigorous exercise plan, which emphasized gradual conditioning through running, walking, and calisthenics, was implemented in some YMCAs. During his career, Cureton achieved some media recognition, but he never attained the celebrity status necessary to create widespread popular awareness of his program.[87]

The YMCA was one organization that addressed men's fitness concerns, but because its branches were locally operated, the quality and type of instruction varied widely. Of the 1,700 Y locations in the United States, at least 100 offered "Business Men's Clubs" (BMCs), which catered to professional white men aged thirty to sixty.[88] Resembling turn-of-the-century athletic clubs, BMCs provided the opportunity to both socialize and exercise (in that order), and prospective members had to undergo an approval process. Membership in most clubs was 99 percent white, with the Harlem Busy Man's Club a notable exception (note the name change—the implication being that black men could not be businessmen). In addition to access to regular Y facilities, such as the swimming pool, BMC members were usually entitled to use a private exercise room that typically included a pulley machine, stationary bicycle, rowing machine, weights, medicine balls, and exercise mats, in addition to handball and squash courts, a nap room, and a lounge.[89] BMC members could also take advantage of the Y's "health service," which offered sauna and steam rooms, ultraviolet and infrared lamps, and massage. Clubs with ambitious fitness directors provided exercise instruction and personalized conditioning programs, but most clubs did not fall into this category. One BMC member described a typical scene at his Cleveland Y:

> Men were sitting in lounge chairs, either sleeping, reading, talking business or discussing politics. Occasionally a man showed up in an athletic suit on his way for some mild exercise, or some member appeared bathed in perspiration. The latter either had played squash, handball or had been working out. Everyone awake would ridicule him and warn him to take it easy. Men came to the Business Men's Club for relaxation, a steam bath, massage, or a quick dip in the pool. This is a typical scene in many BMC's in the country that I've visited.[90]

After being influenced by Cureton, William Cumler, the physical director of the Cleveland Central Branch, instituted a graduated conditioning program consisting of swimming, jogging, and calisthenics. The program's subsequent achievements were considered so groundbreaking that physicians conducted research on members, and journalists reported on the physical feats of exercisers.[91] When one grandfather completed ten miles on the Y track, television, radio, and press reporters covered the event. "Never in its history had Cleveland or any other city seen anything like it. Ten miles—at the age of 63!"[92]

Another initiative instituted in 1963 by many Y locations nationwide was the "Measured Mile" program. Inspired by both Paul Dudley White and John F. Kennedy, the Y and community leaders lobbied local governments for permission to use paint to mark mile-long walking courses on downtown sidewalks. Accounts of the program in small towns indicated that all citizens were invited to walk, but in large cities, the program was specifically targeted to businessmen, who were encouraged to walk a mile during their lunch break. The program was innovative, in that it addressed the lifestyle of middle-class men, and courses were installed in Minneapolis, Boston, Chicago, and New York (where astronaut John Glenn participated in the opening ceremony).[93] Such programs were few, however. Popular and scientific authorities encouraged exercise to prevent heart attacks and to remedy the effects of stressful jobs, but exactly how men were supposed to carry out those recommendations remained unclear through most of the 1960s. Physician input and the expanding consumer health market made it more culturally acceptable to exercise, but American men still lacked specifics. It was this situation that enabled jogging's immediate rise to popularity in the following decade.

For middle-class, white-collar men living in the mid-twentieth century, masculinity was demonstrated through marriage, fatherhood, and gainful employment, not physical prowess or a muscular physique. Beyond a game of golf or touch football, physical activity for self-development was not something most men engaged in or had time for. Even if they were interested in adding exercise to their daily routines, contradictory information made it almost impossible for men to chart a fitness regimen on their own. Physicians' interest in exercising for health had begun to legitimate the pursuit of fitness as a leisure-time habit, but given conflicting opinions on intensity, duration, and suitable activities, it was difficult to know where to begin. As a result, men's hearts often became their wives' responsibility. While this delegation of authority gave women substantial power in the home, it also encouraged men to abdicate responsibility for their own health, creating a pattern with long-term implications. Today, men are much less likely than women to see a physician regularly.[94] The idea that health maintenance is the province of women, a tendency to minimize symptoms, and the belief that willpower can overcome illness all play

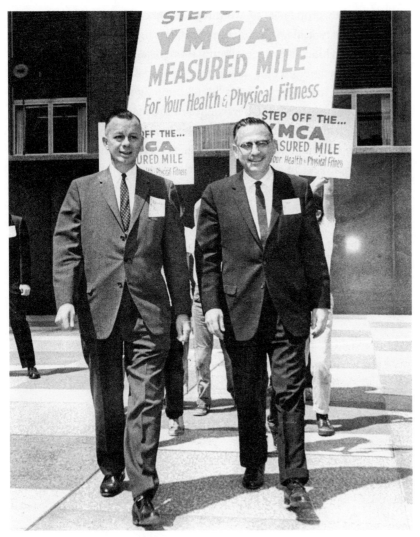

Although the cardiac crisis helped legitimate an interest in exercise, middle-class men had relatively few options for regular physical activity. The YMCA's Measured Mile program, which marked out a mile-long course in the business district of participating towns for lunchtime walks, was one of the few programs adapted to men's lifestyles. In Minneapolis, Mayor Arthur Naftalin (wearing glasses) and his immediate predecessor, Kenneth "PK" Peterson, inaugurated the course in 1963. (Kautz Family YMCA Archives; reprinted by permission of the Minneapolis Star Tribune)

a role in men's propensity to avoid regular checkups as well as more urgent care. The typical heart attack victim has long been characterized as a
professional white male, necessitating more recent campaigns to educate
women and people of color about the dangers of heart disease, such as
the American Heart Association's "Red" campaign. This need for greater
awareness demonstrates the persistence of the idea that heart attacks are
a male problem, when in fact, heart disease is also the leading cause of
death among women. Moreover, the affluence gap that once stemmed the
rate of heart attacks in the African American community no longer holds
true. White and African American men suffer heart attacks at nearly identical rates; however, African Americans suffer higher mortality rates from
heart disease.[95] These trajectories make it clear that cultural perceptions
related to health and disease continue to play a role in popular culture long
after scientific findings have proved them to be outdated. Only by understanding the historical evolution of our beliefs about health and wellness
can contemporary health disparities be resolved.

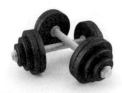

4

In September 1968, a crowd assembled on the National Mall
to celebrate the launch of the National Jogging Association. Founder Richard L. Bohannon, former surgeon general of the air force, was joined by a modest but esteemed
group that included Secretary of the Interior Stewart Udall,
Senator Strom Thurmond (R-S.C.), Representative Henry S.
Reuss (D-Wis.), and Representative Roy A. Taylor (D-N.C.).
Although only a perfunctory 100-yard run had been planned
for the celebration, the energetic assembly joined Bohannon in a quarter-mile jog around the Reflecting Pool. The
recently retired physician imagined that a national association advocating for the concerns of joggers might encourage physical activity among the population at large. Jogging,
Bohannon told the crowd, is the "quickest, cheapest, most
efficient way to achieving physical fitness."[1]

The site of the launch—the Reflecting Pool on the Mall,
situated equidistant from the Lincoln Memorial and the
Washington Monument—seemed to suggest that jogging
had national significance and that physical fitness was a
serious pursuit. This was a marked change from just a few
years earlier, when it had been considered an odd hobby for
middle-class men. Bohannon's status as former surgeon
general of the air force also added importance to the gather-
ing; his backing seemed to imply that jogging was a medi-
cally sound and worthwhile endeavor. The ages of the jog-

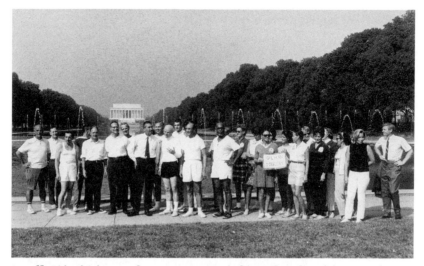

In 1968, Richard Bohannon, former surgeon general of the air force, formed the National Jogging Association to advocate for the needs of joggers. Bohannon, pictured here in black shorts and turtleneck, is flanked by Senator Strom Thurmond (white shorts and T-shirt) and Secretary of the Interior Stewart Udall (dress shirt and tie). Members of the Gilman Joggers, a Baltimore jogging club, were also in attendance. (Collection of Carol Bohannon)

ging dignitaries are also worth noting: Thurmond was the most senior of the group at sixty-five; the other political notables were in their forties and fifties. They were just the type of heart attack–prone men that preventive efforts had been targeting. Bohannon may have thought that such an illustrious assembly would provide inspiration to prospective joggers.

The portrait of this group of joggers challenges popular and scholarly ideas about the kinds of people involved in jogging, their motivations, the timing of the movement, and its origins. Histories of jogging have tended to describe it as a discrete fad, disconnected from the consumer health trends of the 1950s and 1960s, almost as if it had emerged from nothing. Popularly, jogging is often remembered as a "craze" of the 1970s, a fad that appealed to young, long-haired hippies wearing tiny shorts and tube socks, who took to the streets for reasons that had little to do with health.[2] Although this depiction of the typical jogger became more accurate by the second half of the 1970s, the characterization of jogging as a stand-alone fitness phenomenon or the exclusive property of a certain demographic group ignores both the role of health promotion advice in its creation and its first generation of devotees.

The jogging movement of the 1960s and 1970s involved a broad set of interests: health-conscious consumers, politicians of the Left and Right, track athletes, seekers of religion, and former hippies, to name just a few—all of whom imbued their running time with unique significance. Jogging's popularity unfolded in roughly two generations.[3] For middle-aged exercisers who discovered jogging in the mid to late 1960s, their new hobby was a way to cultivate health and still be able to have a steak for dinner. For twenty- and thirty-somethings who discovered jogging after their parents' generation made it popular, it could be a form of self-help, a survivalist technique, a spiritual practice, or a health enhancer—or an amalgam of all four. The "discovery" of jogging by multiple constituencies over time meant that its popularity was continually revived and its appeal reconfigured. The *New York Times* pronounced jogging an "in" sport in 1968, but a decade later, it was still being heralded as the latest trend.[4] That this singular activity was construed as both mainstream and alternative speaks to its malleability and its potential for repurposing and profit making. In the 1970s, jogging became a way of life and a source of personal identity for many people. A closer look at the history of this movement and its trajectory from leisure hobby to lifestyle also reveals the emergence of a new moralism that held individuals entirely accountable for their own health, a problematic idea that continues to pervade contemporary fitness culture.

This chapter is an inclusive (though not necessarily comprehensive) history of the jogging movement. Here, I argue that it is impossible to establish a singular meaning of running or to untangle the disparate motivations that sent Americans to the tracks and trails in the 1960s and 1970s. Even the name of the movement is a case study in subtle difference—*jogging* was the preferred moniker until it was replaced by *running* in the mid-1970s.[5] Jogging effectively functioned as a Rorschach test for the concerns of this era.[6] Throughout the decade, jogging was repeatedly "claimed" by a variety of groups of all political stripes. As both a form of exercise and a statement of solidarity with a host of social concerns, jogging crossed political and cultural lines to become a mass movement. As a preventive health technique, jogging managed to straddle the chasm between traditional medicine and alternative health care. It was this ability to embody a multiplicity of meanings that made it so seductive for advertisers and manufacturers, which promoted jogging and the pursuit of fitness in their messages.

JOGGING'S HEALTH ORIGINS

In 1967, Bill Bowerman, a track coach at the University of Oregon, and W. E. Harris, a cardiologist, published *Jogging*, a slim training manual for nonathletes based on a program Bowerman had devised after working with legendary New Zealand track coach Arthur Lydiard. Lydiard had developed jogging as a way for athletes nearing the end of their competitive years to maintain their physical fitness. Through loosely organized clubs, jogging had become very popular in New Zealand. Bowerman brought Lydiard's ideas back to the United States and organized a jogging club for residents of Eugene, Oregon, in 1963. The popularity of the club—within a month, more than 2,000 joggers of all ages and abilities were attending Bowerman's Sunday sessions—and the wide-ranging fitness levels of its participants convinced the track coach that his program needed medical supervision. After joining forces with Harris, the two ran several small pilot studies to track joggers' health and establish optimal training methods. Jogging clubs quickly spread to other Oregon towns, thanks to the distribution of Harris and Bowerman's booklet *Train . . . Don't Strain*, which they expanded into a book the following year.[7]

Jogging's links to the cardiac crisis were apparent in Bowerman's special handling of former heart attack patients, his association with Harris, and the publicity the program received. Praise for the fitness experiment was widely covered by the national media beginning in 1964.[8] Bowerman and Harris's book recognized adults' lack of opportunity to pursue physical fitness and pointed out that most fitness professionals spent the majority of their time on young people in excellent physical shape, rather than on those who needed their attention the most. The authors listed bowling, hunting, golf, weight lifting, and calisthenics as typical activities among adults who exercised and pointed out that too few were involved in "endurance exercises" that could train the heart, lungs, and circulatory system. *Jogging* provided three twelve-week training schedules for adults in

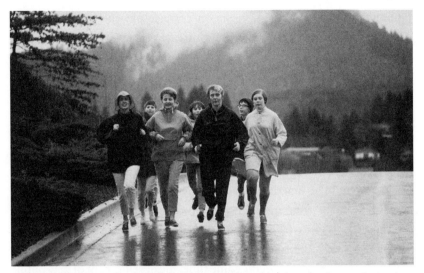

University of Oregon track coach Bill Bowerman popularized jogging when he created a jogging club for Eugene residents in 1963. The group quickly grew to over 2,000 members and led to the publication of Jogging, one of the two books responsible for the jogging movement of the 1970s. This 1969 image of joggers in Eugene illustrates that special clothing and footwear had yet to be mass-marketed. (Photograph by Bates Littlehales, National Geographic, Getty Images)

poor, average, and good condition. Each program stressed the importance of "mak[ing] haste slowly." These recommendations were revolutionary. Unlike competitive sports that demanded an "all-out" level of exertion, a jogging program would be successful and sustainable only if one trained with moderate effort. And unlike once-a-week golf, bowling, or calisthenics, a jogging program required a commitment to exercising at least three times a week for the rest of one's life. In short, following the book's advice meant embarking on a lifestyle change. In return for their efforts, regular joggers could expect improved health and weight loss, as well as increased confidence, an improved outlook, and sexual vigor. Bowerman and Harris's book quickly sold more than a million copies.[9]

On the heels of Jogging, Ken Cooper, another former surgeon general of the air force, published Aerobics in 1968.[10] Based on studies he conducted to improve the fitness of air force personnel, Cooper's book also found instant success. Not unlike Jogging, Aerobics explained in lay terms (although with a greater emphasis on exercise physiology) the benefits of cardiovascular exercise over anaerobic exercise, such as weight lifting, and isometric exercise. Cooper asked readers to test their own physical fitness by measuring how far they could run in twelve minutes. Cooper's book was seminal because he provided an easy-to-grasp definition of *fitness*, a method to gauge one's own fitness level, and an explanation of why cardiovascular fitness was more important than other types. Although Cooper told his readers that swimming and cycling could also provide the benefits of the "training effect," his workout program focused on jogging because it could be practiced anywhere by almost anyone. The book went through fourteen printings, with 2 million copies sold by 1971.[11]

Jogging was also being popularized through the work of Thomas Cureton, whose "Run for Your Life" program was implemented in many YMCAs in the mid-1960s. At the same time, the development of new public spaces promoted jogging. In 1967, the federal government opened four jogging trails on National Park Service property in the Washington, D.C., area. Secretary of the Interior Stewart Udall, accompanied by members of a Baltimore jogging club, inaugurated the Hains Point Trail in East Potomac Park with a two-mile jog. Udall predicted that jogging was "going to catch on nationwide."[12] That same year, U.S. News & World Report estimated that there were already 5 million joggers in the United States.[13] When New York City's Department of Parks opened twenty new jogging trails in 1968, a writer for the Times reported that newcomers were "considerably outnumbered by the experienced joggers," suggesting that jogging had quickly gained a sizable number of participants.[14] Although jogging is most often thought of as a trend of the 1970s, it's clear that it enjoyed substantial popularity in the previous decade and that preventive health awareness was responsible for its cultural ascendance.

The immediate success of jogging can be attributed to the increasing but unchanneled interest in physical fitness, health, and weight loss. As explained in previous chapters, Americans had been admonished to exercise since the mid-1950s, but specifics regarding intensity, duration, and recommended activities were absent, especially for men. In his book, Cooper observed that physicians commonly asked him how to advise patients who inquired about exercise. One doctor admitted encouraging his patients to engage in mild exercise but confided that he never knew how long or how much to recommend.[15] *Jogging* and *Aerobics* each provided specific recommendations and a method to monitor progress. More important, they both advocated a fairly low level of intensity; the challenge of their programs was consistency.

Jogging represented a new kind of physical activity on many levels. It was noncompetitive; in order to win at jogging, one only had to do it regularly. The emphasis on participation over victory was especially attractive to those who did not consider themselves athletic. Instruction books repeatedly emphasized that anyone could become a jogger. As one manual pointed out, "No matter how inadequate you may be as a natural athlete, how little your natural physical endowments may have given you in the way of athletic capability, you can become a good long-distance runner if you have one quality, and that quality is persistence."[16] Success was defined by a healthier heart, a trimmer waistline, and increased endurance—the only failures were people who didn't get up off the couch. Running also differentiated itself from other sports because it encouraged participants to exist in the present, to enjoy training as an end in itself, not as preparation for some future meet or game. It was this quality that later made the practice adaptable by joggers who viewed their time on the track as meditation, prayer, or therapy.

The emphasis on health and on participation regardless of skill level appealed to middle-aged Americans, who had been hearing about new medical research and exercise promotion campaigns for more than a decade and had finally found a way to act on that information. Rather than the baby boomers, who are usually identified as the country's first modern exercisers, it was actually members of the greatest generation who popularized jogging. That it was initially aimed at an older public is clearly visible in early jogging publications and media coverage. Writing in the *New York Times Magazine*, Hal Higdon characterized joggers in 1968 as "securely middle-aged, that great awkward crowd of us too old for LSD and too young for Medicare."[17] When William Zinsser reviewed *Jogging* for *Life* magazine, he doubted the activity would catch on with the younger set.[18] *Time* similarly noted that "the cult of physical fitness has developed into a national middle-aged obsession."[19] The idea that older Americans could and should engage in vigorous exercise was a marked departure from earlier decades, when physical fitness had been cultivated mainly in gym class and varsity sports. "We are subjected to the message that physical achievements end at 25, from which point it is all martinis, divorce and downhill," one older jogger complained.[20] Jogging's vigorous nature also represented a substantial departure from the sedate exercise plans demonstrated on television shows or recommended in earlier health guides.

Despite its almost immediate popularity, exercising in public was still considered something of a novelty through most of the 1960s and 1970s. On the streets, joggers were regarded as oddballs or health nuts at best; they were subjected to harassment and violence at worst. Conflict soon erupted between joggers and drivers; the latter seemed to sense a silent reproach as they sat behind the wheels of their cars. Joggers, for their part, were quick to find virtue in their new habit and resorted to name-calling and judgment of those who hadn't heeded the call to health. As sidewalks and road shoulders filled with runners, each side participated in a heated debate over the appropriate use of public space. Drivers complained that joggers didn't follow the rules of the road or obey traffic signs. One Chicagoan reported that otherwise ordinary citizens were transformed once they put on jogging suits: "these runners in their color-coordinated togs trot down not only the middle of the road but the middle of the sidewalk, the middle of the busy street, and the middle of the intersection as well."[21] A spokesman for the American Automobile Association expressed concern and pointed out that "mixing joggers and cars is dangerous business. The streets are primarily for automobiles."[22] *Road and Track* urged prudence and identified the problem as joggers' ability to behave like both pedestrian and vehicle. "All too often I have witnessed the arrogance of the long-distance runner as he or she takes up an inordinate amount of tarmac and throws traffic safety rules to the wind," the writer asserted.[23]

A number of municipalities considered methods to regulate jogging. A West Chester, Pennsylvania, auto club proposed that the state issue jogging licenses because joggers were hazardous to traffic.[24] The California Motor Vehicle Administration's advisory board also considered a plan to license joggers.[25] The New Jersey senate tried and failed to pass a bill requiring joggers to run on sidewalks and wear reflective clothing at night.[26]

Several towns treated joggers like vehicles, and examples abound of joggers receiving tickets for running red lights (literally!).[27] A few joggers even reported being arrested on various charges while running.[28] In Los Altos Hills, California, home of *Runner's World* magazine, large groups of runners regularly occupied the full width of roads on Sundays, inciting the city council to hold a series of meetings on whether to ban jogging within city limits.[29] David Proft, sponsor of a proposed ordinance to outlaw groups of two or more runners on local roads, complained that runners "swarm around your car like locusts."[30]

Besides traffic circulation and safety issues, some authorities worried that the sight of large numbers of exercisers might be unseemly. When residents of Annapolis, Maryland, complained that groups of jogging midshipmen from the Naval Academy disturbed the tranquility of the town, jogging routes were restricted.[31] In an effort to curb the number of men running shirtless, the town of Palm Beach, Florida, banned bare chests outside the beach area in 1981—the second year in a row the town council had enacted such legislation. The previous year, lawyers for the 1,000-member Palm Beach Runners' Association had successfully challenged the ordinance, which a court found unconstitutional. Fearing "an invasion of topless joggers" protesting the new law, police refused to say when they would start to enforce the ban.[32] Officials at Arlington National Cemetery also began to enforce a policy that prohibited jogging on the grounds. "Joggers are just running through there all the time and it doesn't look very good," one military official complained. Yet as protesting joggers pointed out, they were free to walk through the grounds; only jogging was being targeted.[33]

For their part, runners regularly reported poor treatment at the hands of motorists, including being chased off the road, shouted at, and having objects thrown at them from cars, even during races. Female runners were often the object of jeers and catcalls.[34] Fed up, runners gradually became adamant about their right to use the streets. They fought back against drivers who didn't share the roads and made obscene gestures, heckled those who threw objects, and even trampled the hoods of cars when drivers failed to respect crosswalks.[35] One group of runners in New York's Central Park reportedly attacked a taxi that violated weekend vehicle restrictions.[36]

With few dedicated spaces of their own, runners were forced to create their own trails. "Until there are enough safe running paths, we'll keep fighting for our constitutional right to use the roads," one jogger testified in Los Altos Hills.[37]

The mutual antipathy between joggers and motorists hinted at a new and increasing sense of moralism in exercise discourse. Joggers speculated that they were the object of hostility because the sight of them forced nonrunners to confront their own inactivity. Runners believed that their sense of healthiness and well-being, which only those involved in vigorous exercise could know, distinguished them from nonrunners. In 1968, *New York Times* sportswriter Robert Lipsyte pointed out the psychic changes that are the by-products of a faithful exercise routine: "The hobbyist-athlete gains that edge, that hard righteousness of sacrifice and superiority that is not only insufferable to fat smokers, but scares them."[38] One runner-writer for the *Los Angeles Times* similarly surmised that runners "can represent an affront to the sedentary person, who might well drop dead if he tried to keep up the pace for even one block."[39]

The regularity of a jogging routine engendered a new kind of personal identity grounded in a commitment to health and self. One commentator suggested that this identity was a result of the sense of achievement from completing a daily jog, as well as the potential for unlimited improvement in distance or speed.[40] Running journalists seemed to agree that an air of moral superiority was a natural by-product of a jogging regimen. "Joggers and runners are part of an elite. You cannot keep this up for more than six or eight months of time before you begin to feel, 'I'm a better person than someone who is not doing this sport,'" Hal Higdon noted in a 1976 *Runner's World* article.[41]

Maintaining a healthy body and living an active life were central to the running identity. Joggers' sense of supremacy came as much from what they didn't do as from what they did. Their disregard for the rules of the road may have been linked to their perception that drivers were sedentary, overeating, cigarette-addicted polluters. One *Runner's World* writer imagined (hoped?) how she and a friend looked to others:

On a hot, muggy day in Washington, DC, two runners go steaming up the middle of traffic clogged Wisconsin Avenue, flaunting the fact that they aren't tied to a dull desk job. Out-of-shape businessmen on their way to three-martini lunches, forced to slam on their brakes to avoid hitting them, are doubly perturbed. Not only does it frazzle their nerves like any other traffic nuisance—they also know deep down that they should be out doing the very same thing.[42]

Running publications had no prohibitions on name-calling. In *Runner's World*, David Zinman labeled his nonrunning neighbors "fatty-pies and smokers and gone-to-paunch sportsmen."[43] The new sense of righteousness that accompanied a regular jogging regimen was a marked difference from the casual attitudes that had characterized setting-up exercises and television workouts in earlier decades. It was evident that one's exercise routine as well as one's health were matters to be taken seriously, and those who did not exercise could be considered deviant.

THE NATURAL LIFE

For the contingent of joggers who took up the activity in the 1960s, jogging represented a way to maintain one's lifestyle in a more healthful fashion. The underlying goal of jogging, as it was outlined by Bowerman, Harris, and Cooper, was to mitigate the perils of civilization. To that end, it was not so different from the Cold War calisthenics intended to keep children strong while allowing them to indulge in the abundance of the postwar economy. The introduction to *Jogging*, for example, referenced the midcentury complaint that Americans of the past had been hardier, pointing out that New Zealanders who jogged "were possessed of the same vigor that characterized Americans 50 years ago."[44] Richard Bohannon, in his introduction to *Aerobics*, also echoed earlier charges that a modern existence did not provide the necessary physical exertion: "In this age of mechanization and automation, we know that our normal work activities do not provide the exercise our bodies, our muscles, and our hearts and lungs require."[45]

For the second, generally younger contingent of joggers, who became involved after jogging had achieved a measure of popularity in the 1970s, running was exercise, but it could also function as a political statement, a rite of environmental solidarity, or an expression of disapproval of an unhealthy world. Second-generation joggers believed that running allowed them to return to a more natural state—one that would have occurred spontaneously if not for the effects of living in a man-made world. This reworked critique of consumption and abundance echoed earlier laments of a utopian past that had required more of one's physical body, but at the same time, it reflected decidedly 1970s-era environmental concerns.

Proponents claimed that running was an activity all humans knew how to do instinctively. "The procedure of running is simplicity itself. There are no lessons, no gurus, no equipment, no right way, no wrong way," one *Runner's World* contributor wrote.[46] Authors of running manuals often noted that modern-day joggers were reconnecting with the Greeks, prehistoric hunter-gatherers, preindustrial laborers, or other "natural" peoples. The author of *Return to Running* included an entire history of evolution in his manual, illustrating his belief that early humanoids were runners.[47] The Tarahumara Indians of Mexico, for whom long-distance running is a rite of passage, were also frequently cited as evidence that running is a natural exercise.[48]

Much like the push-button gadgets blamed in earlier decades, Americans now pointed the finger at "machines" for their inactivity and unhealthy lifestyles. According to joggers, machines prevented the human body from engaging in "natural" activities. The text of a 1978 Nike ad drove home this point: "When it comes to making our lives easier, machines have really done a good job. Maybe too good. Machines save us so much work, they've actually put our bodies out of a job. They're killing us. But runners are bringing this country back to life again. . . . To some of us, running is a way of life. . . . Machines can't run."[49]

The most obvious symbol of the power of machines was the car. Earlier critics had made the same point in their condemnation of the new automobility required by suburbia, but the problem was no longer seen in relation to housing. Instead, in line with the decade's environmental turn, cars were demonized for their reliance on fossil fuels, the dependence they encouraged in humans, and the pollution they spewed.[50] The debate over joggers' right to use the roads was also a demonstration of this animosity toward the automobile.

Persistent gas shortages during the decade gave runners an opportunity to assert their special ability to withstand hardship and distance themselves from a reliance on cars. *Runner's World* told readers that being physically fit would prepare them for the next gas shortage: "Runners . . . can lead the campaign to revive the almost extinct pair of legs that adorn the human species. This oil shortage could be the impetus we've needed to get people to use that long neglected source of energy—the human body. The time is approaching when runners will be considered as prophets who long ago began preparing for the oil shortage."[51] A 1979 Nike ad illustrated the same idea: A runner sprints past a Texaco gas station with "No Gas" signs pasted to the front window and pumps. The caption, "A Bit of Independence," refers to the runner's own ability as well as his freedom from the vagaries of Middle Eastern oil supplies.[52]

Worries about fossil fuel depletion were part of a larger concern about the environment in general. The fact that runners normally exercised outdoors heightened their sensitivity to pollution issues. Running publications carried articles about the potential dangers of jogging in traffic, which meant breathing in smog and exhaust fumes, and they were often sympathetic with environmental concerns, stressing that runners were more in tune with nature.[53] Running also intersected with a growing belief in the need for self-sufficiency and the interest in survivalism, which was related to the environmental movement and a lack of faith in the establishment. Publications such as *Mother Jones* and the *Whole Earth Catalog* were part of a trend to educate Americans how to withstand a time when, as some predicted, government broke down and food stores were empty.[54] The growing interest in home gardening and solar energy wasn't fueled only by concerns about the environment—the self-sufficiency of living off the electrical grid and supplying one's own food was part of the attraction. Running provided a similar independence in the form of a high-functioning body and a sense of personal autonomy. One long-winded subscription advertisement for *Running Times* spotlighted these concerns: "We have begun to discover that our real strength is not in our government, our economy, or our property but in ourselves. Through our running, we are discovering the joys of a personal sufficiency and fitness for life that we never dreamed of ten or twenty years ago."[55] As a form of travel that was not dependent on fossil fuels, running functioned as a survival tactic. Some runners imagined their training as preparation for an era when legs, not cars, would be the primary mode of transportation.

One runner expressed the hope that drive-through bank and restaurant windows would someday be replaced by run-up windows.[56]

During the 1970s, a bevy of books encouraged Americans to reform their domestic habits for the improvement of the world as a whole. Barry Commoner's *The Closing Circle* (1972), E. F. Schumacher's *Small Is Beautiful* (1973), Paul Ehrlich's *The End of Affluence* (1974), and Frances Moore Lappé's *Diet for a Small Planet* (1975) made it clear that the United States was only one player in a global economy, while highlighting the fact that individual efforts could have global repercussions.[57] The interconnectedness between Americans and others was often demonstrated through ordinary activities imbued with tremendous political significance. One's diet, for example, could function as a political statement. In the 1970s, fasting, embracing vegetarianism, eating a macrobiotic diet, and shopping at natural food stores and food co-ops were popular ways to show allegiance to environmental causes and protest world hunger.[58] Running was a similar gesture; its practitioners, however, were painfully aware of the pointlessness of their acts. One new convert to running concluded that the phenomenon had been "brought on, to a significant degree, by a sense of frustration. . . . Somehow the idea of being able to run a mile or two farther every month or so was probably subconsciously more appealing than trying but continually failing to solve the problems of the poor and oppressed." At least, he quipped, protesters in the 1980s would likely be too quick for the police to catch them.[59]

The notion that some joggers were acting in support of issues beyond their own immediate health concerns challenges the oft-repeated charge that Americans of the 1970s were narcissistic and self-absorbed. Critics such as Christopher Lasch, who portrayed the nation's citizens as inward looking to the point of "navel gazing," argued that running (among other activities) indicated that Americans no longer cared about political change.[60] In fact, the opposite is true. Jogging should be viewed as one of many cultural movements, such as feminism and environmentalism, that linked the personal with the political. Historian Peter Filene has called running and other fitness pursuits of the 1970s "a private version of the ecology movement," which helps explain how jogging resonated with citizens who were concerned about both health and environmental issues.[61]

One jogger also made this linkage, attributing the running phenomenon to the desire to take action but the ability to act only on the terrain closest at hand—the self: "We feel more or less helpless and yet, at the same time, desirous to protect what resources we can. We . . . protect our nearest natural resource—our physical health—in the almost superstitious hope that such small gestures will help save an earth that we are blighting."[62]

JOGGING AS SELF-HELP

Feeling better had always been an advertised by-product of a jogging regimen, but the magnitude of that claim increased dramatically during the 1970s, which also saw a renewed interest in mental health therapeutics. Runners believed their routines could cure mental health problems, curtail addictive behavior, or even deepen their relationship with God. Although research has shown that exercise can alleviate the symptoms of depression, the extravagant claims of some running promoters seem more representative of the decade's preoccupations rather than jogging's ability to heal. This tendency to view exercise as a panacea continued a trend that Jack La Lanne and a few others had initiated in the 1960s—associating exercise with positive internal qualities, such as a happy disposition or professional competency. Beginning with Bowerman, Harris, and Cooper, experts had promised that running would make one feel better and improve one's general disposition, but some enthusiasts made wide-reaching claims that running could change one's total outlook on life. The authors of *Keep Your Heart Running* informed readers that after a jog, "the feeling of well-being will make boring tasks possible to tolerate with a laugh, and work that we like will become a joy."[63] Even health-focused manuals, such as *The Joy of Jogging*, made significant claims about running's potential to improve one's life, promising that "a blighted, boring life can become luminous and glorious under the beat, beat, beat of a heart rejuvenated by the joys of jogging."[64]

Claims about running's nontangible effects grew increasingly grandiose as the decade wore on. By the late 1970s, nearly all running manuals promised a wonderful feeling of well-being and euphoria that began about halfway into one's run. Calling it a runner's high, the media likened this state to a drug-induced high. *House and Garden* informed readers, "Running has the same effect as drugs. You get a high and don't want to stop."[65] Nike also perpetuated the mystique and exclusivity of the runner's high in print ads, calling it "a special, very personal experience that is unknown to most people. Some call it euphoria. Others say it's a new kind of mystical experience that propels you into an elevated state of consciousness. A flash of joy. A sense of floating as you run."[66] Even for those with no interest in fitness, these claims likely made nonrunners curious about what they were missing, perhaps inspiring a jog in the park. Not surprisingly, the press tended to gloss over the actual hard labor of running.

Other runners, especially those with competitive track backgrounds or who ran primarily for health reasons, expressed doubt about these claims. According to one skeptical runner, a runner's high was "only experienced by those runners who live in California."[67] One reader wrote to congratulate *Running Times* on an article that cast doubt on the phenomenon, explaining, "The most I have ever experienced is the pleasure of feeling my body in motion and an appreciation of the sometimes beautiful scenery. I do not doubt that the runner's high exists, merely that it is not all that it is cracked up to be."[68] Running legend Walt Stack agreed: "Once in a while a sort of euphoric feeling envelops me when I reach the last few miles homeward. But usually the only high I get is from fantasizing while following one of our faster running sisters."[69]

The runner's high hype was emblematic of why many younger runners took to the streets. Rather than preventing heart attacks or lowering cholesterol, second-generation joggers were interested, above all, in having an intense experience. Running made exhaustion more profound, happiness more euphoric, sensation more vivid. Because jogging provided an opportunity to think freely and largely uninterrupted for a length of time, it's not surprising that some runners saw their outings as occasions to commune with a higher being. Turning running into a spiritual practice was in line with the decade's surge in religiosity. Evangelicalism and new religious movements characterized the 1970s. Books such as *Zen Running*, *The Zen of Running*, *Holistic Running*, and *Beyond Jogging: The Innerspaces of Running* showed runners how to turn their exercise routines into a mode of worship.[70] Specialty magazines frequently discussed the religious qualities of running: in its regularity, running was a ritual; the process by which one became a runner was often referred to in terms of conversion; and the outdoor nature of the run put runners in God's own church.[71] Joel Henning's appreciation of his regular jog illustrates the spirituality of his running practice:

> I am a runner. Four or five mornings a week I awake at 6:00 a.m., anoint my feet with Vaseline or tincture of benzoin or powder (or all three), cover my worst blisters with tape, and approach the jumble of sweat clothes, athletic socks, shorts, and mottled jockstrap that is draped over the portable TV in my bedroom, as if it were a primitive altar. In fact, it is the symbol of a kind of worship involving holy breathing, obtestation, propitiation, atonement, sacrifice, exorcism, karma, *asanas*, and meditation.[72]

It wasn't only seekers of nontraditional religious experiences who saw running as an opportunity for quiet thought and meditation. White middle-class Christians, especially Protestants, accounted for the majority of joggers, and they too explored how a running habit could be integrated into their religious lives. Echoing the biblical command that believers should make their bodies a temple for the Lord, authors of mainstream religious running books explained how running could be an integral part of a Christian life. According to books such as *Jog for Your Life* and *Running the Race: The Spiritual Benefits of Running*, a religious purpose could be the motivating factor in a decision to begin or continue a jogging regimen.[73] "Make your jogging program a spiritual program growing out of your love for the Lord," Ted Frederick suggested. He reminded readers that "the Lord Jesus Christ chose a life of physical activity" and that Peter "was no slouch in the physical fitness department."[74]

When the results of an exercise regimen led to the confidence to make changes in other aspects of life, running became a therapeutic technique. Similar to other 1970s trends such as biofeedback, Esalen, Erhard seminars, and transcendental meditation, jogging appealed to those searching for ways to perfect the self. Because it promised both physical and mental rehabilitation, jogging had more to offer than therapies involving the mind alone. The belief that a jogging habit could transform one's life may have been the inspiration for many runners of the 1970s.

Films of the decade reinforced the notion that jogging could change lives. The 1978 TV movie *See How She Runs* advanced the idea of running as self-help: Betty Quinn, an unfulfilled geography teacher, only dreams about the exotic locales she discusses in class. Quinn, played by Joanne Woodward (who won an Emmy for her performance), is a single mother and a new jogging convert whose decision to run in the Boston Marathon ultimately gives her the confidence to make other positive changes in her life. When Quinn confides to a colleague about her plan, her colleague speculates that running may be a way to "get back a little," telling Quinn that she has been "giving [her]self away for a long time now." Quinn's running parallels other positive changes in her personal life. When Quinn's training regimen takes time away from her daughters, they must learn to accept that she has interests independent of motherhood, and consequently, they learn to treat her with more respect. As she embarks on longer runs, Quinn takes more risks, choosing to reject a reconciliation proposal from her ex-husband (and the financial security it would bring) and lecturing her children that it is far worse "never to be scared" than to be afraid. After the race, the film hints, Quinn will realize her dream of traveling the foreign rivers she has previously only described to her class.

The film's real story is that the character's personal development is made possible by running. Quinn's positive life changes are depicted as far more important than the race itself. On the day of the marathon, midway through the course, Quinn develops cramps and slows to a walk. When she finally finishes the race, stumbling in pain and dead last, night is falling and the route has already been reopened to cars. But the sound track's triumphant music and the family and friends awaiting her arrival make it clear that she is a winner. In line with jogging's emphasis on participation rather than victory, the film demonstrates that running the race is nowhere near as important as preparing for it. Viewers are expected to discern that the physical training of the jogging regimen has taught Quinn confidence, perseverance, and inner strength. The pain she feels is clear, but her ability to complete the race demonstrates a new self-mastery that will translate to other parts of her personal life. With the knowledge that she has completed a marathon, she can do anything.[75]

Running proponents argued that in addition to curing low self-esteem, a running routine could treat more serious forms of psychological trauma and even mental illness. A Vietnam veteran told readers of Runner's World that running had helped him overcome what would now be diagnosed as post-traumatic stress disorder.[76] An alcoholic attested that running had helped him stop drinking.[77] Running was also frequently discussed as rehabilitative therapy for prison inmates. Running magazines occasionally ran reports filed by inmates on the running conditions at various prisons and on the exercise routines they maintained while incarcerated.[78] The ABC movie The Jericho Mile, which recounted the story of a marathon run behind prison walls, further popularized the notion that running was therapeutic.[79]

By 1976, there were at least two books on the market that promoted running as a cure for mental illness, and one psychologist had started an organization for therapists who used running in their practices.[80] In his book Positive Addiction, psychiatrist William Glasser suggested that addictions to drugs, gambling, and alcohol, as well as general malaise, could be overcome by replacing "negative addictions" with positive ones. Glasser theorized that certain activities such as running and meditation had the power to induce a state of mental creativity and confidence that rendered their practitioners strong and thus able to overcome their problems. As Glasser saw it, we "choose the misery in our lives," and sheer strength of will could overcome these problems.[81] In a similar vein, psychiatrist Thaddeus Kostrubala, who had undergone a personal transformation after taking up running for health reasons, realized that a running regimen might also be beneficial for the patients he saw in group therapy. After working with three groups of patient-runners, Kostrubala determined that a running session followed by a therapy session was highly beneficial, even for patients suffering from schizophrenia. He went so far as to predict that running therapy would become an established form of psychotherapy.[82]

In 1978, running hype reached its apotheosis with the publication of Valerie Andrews's The Psychic Power of Running, which included chapters on how running could alleviate depression, help cure cancer, ensure business success, make women more assertive, function as a form of moving meditation, and "unravel the mysteries of the unconscious," all in a slim 165-page paperback.[83] Works like this, along with incessant media coverage and the self-satisfied smugness of some runners, resulted in a backlash by those who couldn't bear to hear another word about running's restorative powers. Frank Deford, a writer at *Sports Illustrated*, summed up the feelings of many when he complained in 1978:

> I am sick of joggers and I am sick of runners. I don't care if all the people in the US are running or are planning to run or wish they could run. . . . I don't ever again want to read about the joy of running, the beauty, the ecstasy, the pain, the anguish, the agony, the rapture, the enchantment, the thrill, the majesty, the love, the coming-togetherness, the where-it's-at-ness. I don't ever again want to hear running compared to religion, sex, or ultimate truth.[84]

While some, such as the authors of *The Non-Runner's Book* (whose red cover poked fun at Jim Fixx's best seller), used humor to make their point, serious runners found nothing funny about antirunning sentiment.[85] Runner-writer Colman McCarthy reported on the backlash and warned runners to "stop running off at the mouth about [running]."[86] Even Fixx intervened in the debate, urging runners to put a stop to some of the movement's most elevated claims, charging that "this sort of windy hyperbole is just plain silly."[87]

THE BUSINESS OF RUNNING

Running's ability to be imbued with any kind of meaning represented an irresistible opportunity for marketers and manufacturers to sell not only jogging products but any item that could be linked with exercise or a healthy lifestyle. Second-generation joggers in particular, who viewed running as a form of cultural critique, were scandalized when the jogging world transitioned from subculture to mass culture. What had once been touted as a free-to-all activity soon required a full complement of gear.

As early as 1968, manufacturers began to market accessories specifically designed for joggers. Good shoes were, of course, the first item a novice jogger purchased, and an increasing number of manufacturers and retail outlets sprang up to cater to that market.[88] Sporting goods chains were expanding rapidly, and manufacturers tried to distinguish their products with technical design improvements. By 1979, running shoes were a $500 million business.[89] Must-have accessories soon included skin lubricant, key pouches, orthotic shoe inserts, and stopwatches, among other items. A cartoon in the National Jogging Association's newsletter the *Jogger* depicted one gear-laden man lamenting to another, "By the time I changed into my custom jogging suit, strapped on my pedometer, portable radio, heart monitor, and slipped into my special jogging shoes it was too late to go out and jog![90] Fashion-forward workout clothing, especially two-piece warm-up suits in bright colors, became de rigueur not only for jogging but for any activity, making jogging apparel the first athletic clothing to gain acceptance as casual wear. That fashion and sport intersected to such an extent illustrated the breadth of the movement.[91] "Manufacturers have overcome all obstacles and made running big business," attested one runner with a complete running wardrobe.[92] This situation seemed far removed from jogging in the late 1960s. The photos in Bowerman and Harris's *Jogging* featured sixty-something matrons circling the track in trench coats and plastic rain scarves, while their male counterparts were clad in button-down shirts, khaki pants, and belts.[93]

Like the sale of running gear, the publication of how-to guides for runners became a profitable business by the late 1970s.[94] In addition to general guides for new runners, there were health- and spirituality-oriented volumes, training manuals for marathoners, guides for traveling runners, and biographies of famous runners. *Runner's World*, the best-known running magazine, saw its circulation increase from 500 in 1968 to 500,000 by 1979, and the new titles *Running Times* and the *Runner* challenged its domination of the periodical market.[95]

As the number of runners increased, so did interest in road racing. Both the number of participants and the number of races soared over the course of the 1970s. San Francisco's eight-mile Bay to Breakers race, for example, grew from 292 participants in 1966 to 8,861 runners in 1977, which didn't include several thousand unregistered "bandits."[96] Used to relatively quiet affairs, race organizers found it increasingly difficult to handle so many runners, the majority of whom participated to validate their weekly jogging regimens, commune with other like-minded individuals, and compete against their own best times, rather than win. Many race directors accepted commercial sponsorships as a way to control the rising costs of bigger races. New York Road Runners Club (NYRRC) president Fred Lebow admitted that pleasing both sponsors and runners was difficult: "We are walking a tightrope balanced between runners' being used by the sponsors and what the sponsors should get out of it."[97] One article in *Advertising Age*, referring to the logo-laden T-shirts that were rapidly becoming a standard perk of the race entry fee, encouraged businesses to consider "these mercurial messengers not as health nuts but as a resource of 20,000,000 or so miniature migratory billboards."[98] Some runners, however, objected to the increasing collusion between running and big business. They took exception to the presence of advertising on the race numbers they were assigned to wear and to race entry forms that required them to consent to the use of their images in advertisements.[99]

In particular, runners resented the linking of unhealthy products with the running lifestyle through race sponsorship. Cardiologist George Sheehan, a noted running author and running's chief metaphysical guru, became the spokesman for Anheuser-Busch Natural Light beer after an anecdote circulated that he had consumed five beers during the 1977 Boston Marathon. Sheehan authored an instructional booklet on running distributed in conjunction with an ad campaign entitled "Run Like a Natural," which linked running to the "natural" beer. The brand sponsored races throughout the country and awarded completion certificates containing the beer's logo to participants, including children and teens, which angered health-oriented joggers.[100]

Jim Fixx, author of *The Complete Book of Running* and the national authority on running, drew runners' ire when he appeared at a series of ten-kilometer races sponsored by Quaker Natural Cereal called the 100% Natural Runs. At one San Francisco race, 250 protesters demonstrated against the "overcommercialization" of running and Quaker's health claims about its cereal, which was 21 percent sugar. One protester charged, "The time has come for runners to speak out and tell Quaker and other corporations which follow its example that we will boycott races which subsidize the advertising of unwholesome products under the guise of being a public service."[101] Runners became outraged when Fixx continued to cash in on the fame resulting from his book. One irate runner wrote an open letter to Fixx in *Running Times*, castigating him for the profit-seeking motives behind his promotion of a credit card and a soft drink. Paul Kiell wasn't angry that Fixx had appeared in the ads; he was angry that the products Fixx endorsed were contrary to a running philosophy that embraced a lifestyle of simplicity:

> First you did it when you were featured in a commercial promoting a principle that you can have what you want, when you want it, immediately by the mere use of a credit card. Not really that bad, but then you did one of a soft drink, its purveyors attempting to associate themselves with running, with you as their symbol. That did it. You had an opportunity to set an example and get a totally different message across to the American public. At the very least you could have kept silent, and not lent your good name to the wolves.[102]

Kiell's letter highlights the contrast between the first and second generations of runners. For Kiell, running included believing in a set of principles that embraced a holistic approach to health and an anticonsumption mentality.

For Fixx, a magazine editor who had started running for health reasons in 1968 and was thus part of jogging's first generation, running was primarily exercise.[103] Although *The Complete Book of Running* discussed the mind-body connection, Fixx concentrated mainly on the technical aspects of running, such as how to train and what to wear. Some runners were scandalized by Fixx's attitude, but his actions were not surprising. Many runners with similar backgrounds also failed to see the changes brought about by running's growing popularity as a loss of purity. Runners who had lived through the early years—when they were considered kooks, had few races to participate in, and could not find good shoes or specialized clothing—were not nostalgic for the past.[104] Before the mid-1970s, other than shoes and track suits, necessities such as sports bras could be acquired only by mail order from specialty companies that advertised in the back pages of running magazines. In 1974, runner Janet Heinonen joked that finding running apparel for women was "as easy as finding gasoline on the weekend."[105] After attending a sporting goods show in the late 1970s, the publisher of *Runner's World* reminded readers that they were lucky to have so many footwear options, noting, "It wasn't too long ago that this was not the case."[106] As late as 1977, one runner, unable to find waterproof gear, happily reported that plastic garbage bags did a great job protecting his cotton sweat suit during rainstorms.[107]

While the increasingly commercial nature of running had both positive and negative aspects, it was running insiders themselves who sought to increase the number of participants in road races and, by extension, the number of runners overall. In her study of the New York Marathon, historian Pamela Cooper suggests that by gradually extending the time allowed to complete the race, organizers served the needs of corporate sponsors by increasing the number of runners, and thus the number of consumers, exposed to their brands. Before the arrival of fitness runners on the racing scene, marathon organizers typically closed the course after four hours, and the finish times of the slowest runners were not recorded. The influence of health-oriented jogging on competitive running led to awards for all finishers and a race course that remained open longer. Cooper argues that the organizer of the race, the NYRRC, delivered to sponsors a privileged market demographic that the club cultivated in order to expand its power base and generate revenue.[108] Cooper's work shows that although running magazines and academics had long documented that the majority of joggers were middle- and upper-class white males (and, later in the decade, females), those involved in running promotion also catered to this group, thereby enhancing the self-selecting effect.

Women's growing involvement in running was affected by the same market forces driving racing in general. Although increasing the number of female runners was a commendable goal, it was also commercially desirable for promoters, because women represented a relatively untapped market. To help increase women's participation in races, Lebow and the NYRRC organized what would become an annual event—a women-only ten-kilometer race (then referred to as a mini-marathon) sponsored by the manufacturer of a women's shaving cream. The club avidly promoted the race, handing out flyers and taping them to light poles. Publicity promoted not only the race and its sponsors but also the NYRRC and running in general, further enlarging the running public and the club's potential constituency.[109]

Single-sex events helped encourage female joggers to formalize their participation and validated their athletic status. Women who became involved in the jogging movement often had no experience in fitness pursuits beyond high school gym class, and for many, running represented a first encounter with the power of their bodies. As one woman put it, running provided "an understanding of myself not only as intellect and soul, but also body."[110] By 1977, it was estimated that more than 500,000 women ran or jogged regularly, up from 25,000 in 1972.[111] In spite of gains made by the women's movement and Title IX, female runners still had to contend with several barriers during the 1970s. The myth that women's bodies couldn't handle long distances, the notion that vigorous exercise was unfeminine, child-care issues, a lack of appropriate apparel, and exclusion from some races continued to present obstacles.[112]

As the jogging movement and the feminist movement unfolded at roughly the same time, some female joggers imagined their exercise regimens as an expression of their growing self-knowledge and power. Changing bodies became a point of pride. One *Redbook* contributor described changes that went beyond an improved appearance:

> I noted that my legs had developed a more muscular look and that gave me a curious feeling of elation. The new muscles symbolized for me a new kind of beauty—the beauty of accomplishment rather than of decoration. I had grown up in a family in which it was most important that a girl be "ladylike" and to be ladylike was to remain unruffled and cool. The very antithesis of a lady was someone who sweated or developed muscles. In short, ladies were spectators.[113]

While some women found it impossible to maintain a running program because of demands on their time from husbands and children, others used running to legitimate spending time on themselves. A mother of quadruplets switched her exercise routine from tennis to running because "I just had to make time to get out of the house and away from the children every day. . . . I needed time for myself."[114] Likewise, another mother who initially felt guilty about running came to believe that it was time well spent: "Gradually, I have come to realize that by developing myself through running, becoming a happier, more fulfilled person, I am helping my children. Running and raising a family can, and do, go well together."[115]

While the running world took steps to increase the number of runners overall, and women constituted a large part of that effort, Americans of color remained a slim percentage of joggers throughout the 1970s. African American newspapers reported on the new exercise, the establishment of local jogging clubs, and the development of trails and parks, but to a lesser degree than other publications. In addition, many of these articles were wire reports rather than pieces written specifically for the African American community. YMCAs in predominantly African American communities did promote jogging as a part of a national initiative. The Harlem YMCA, for example, started a jogging club in 1968. It met three times a week and followed Thomas Cureton's Run for Your Life program. The following year, 200 Harlem joggers took part in a program to complete 125 miles over 25 weeks to celebrate the Y's 125th anniversary.[116] Data on African American participation in running are scant. Although African Americans certainly participated in jogging as a leisure activity, they did so at a much lower level than the overall population. According to one estimate, blacks constituted only 1 to 3 percent of all racers in the New York Marathon.[117]

One obstacle to African American participation in jogging may have been a lack of safe public spaces to train. In the early years, most joggers were forced to contend with taunts from drivers, but black runners faced particularly harsh conditions. In 1971, runner Lou Scott complained, "I'll be running along and a car will come alongside me. The cat inside will roll down the window and I know what he's going to say. 'N——!'"[118] The racist assumption that an African American jogger might be fleeing, possibly from a crime, has long plagued black men. Even in the twenty-first century, one young African American listed "don't run in public" as one of the rules for black men learning to negotiate white culture.[119]

White runners occasionally expressed surprise at the sight of black runners, based on a racist stereotype that African Americans were incapable of running long distances and were only capable sprinters.[120] This view, which applied to both leisure and sports running, derived from the belief that victory in longer races depended on strategy and training. Short-distance runners, in contrast, were said to win because of sheer physical ability. Scholars have documented the tendency to attribute the athletic success of people of color to "natural" ability rather than hard work or intelligent strategizing.[121] This stereotype held sway even as African Americans made inroads in running for sport and recreation. In the mid-1950s and 1960s, for example, marathoner Ted Corbitt, who founded and was the first president of the Road Runners Club of America and the New York Road Runners Club, was a seminal figure in the development of long-distance road racing.[122]

One black jogger, New York sportswriter Bill Lewis, attributed the comparative lack of interest in the African American community to the fact that long-distance running provided few professional remunerative opportunities, failing to offer young people "a way out of Harlem or Bed-Stuy." Some African Americans resisted the belief that the low participation rate in the black community was related to race, seeing it more as a function of class. According to one Washington radio broadcaster, items such as magazine subscriptions and race entry fees, which could be used to gauge participation, may have been prohibitively expensive for some black runners, thereby creating artificially low participation statistics. Lewis noted a gradual increase in fellow black participants at races over the course of the 1970s, observing, "The proportion of blacks running is about the same as the proportion of middle class or black professionals."[123] Media coverage of African American celebrities points to rising interest in jogging near the end of the decade. Ebony and Jet frequently ran features on the lifestyles of actors, musicians, and politicians, many of whom cited jogging as a hobby in articles published after 1976. Eartha Kitt, Cicely Tyson, Newark mayor Kenneth Gibson, and comedian and activist Dick Gregory were among African American notables who jogged. Both publications occasionally addressed jogging-related health issues, but again, only near the end of the decade.[124]

Throughout the 1970s and into the following decade, running was perceived as a hobby of the white middle and upper classes. Joggers were typically described as white-collar, well-educated nonsmokers, and this perception was supported by numerous surveys taken by running organizations and publications.[125] Working-class Americans often expressed bemusement or disdain of runners and their habit. *Runner's World* columnist Joe Henderson described returning to his native Iowa, where running was considered an oddity by the farmers there. According to his brother-in-law, "Running is a middle- and upper-class luxury. The people who do it are the ones with good jobs, good incomes and time on their hands. The people here (in Iowa farming towns) have to scrape for a living. They can't waste any of their effort on anything as frivolous as sports."[126] Both the late arrival of jogging in the larger African American community and its absence from rural and working-class environments indicate a lack of penetration of preventive health information in populations other than the middle and upper classes and demonstrate just how noninclusive those early information campaigns were.

THE COST OF GOOD HEALTH

The speed with which jogging became a national movement, as well as its origins as a health therapy, might lead one to believe that medical authorities agreed that vigorous exercise was beneficial to heart health. But in spite of all the training manuals, media attention, and word-of-mouth notoriety, debate continued throughout the decade whether jogging was actually good for one's health. Although a majority of the public seemed to believe that exercise in general, and running specifically, was beneficial—or at least not harmful—some physicians were slow to agree. Research had established that exercise could help strengthen the circulatory system, clear cholesterol from the body, and lower blood pressure, but it had not been proved to extend one's life span or prevent heart disease.[127] Many doctors remained skeptical of the health benefits of exercise, and the medical literature of the era repeatedly emphasized the need for additional research.[128]

A number of physicians, however, had already made up their minds about the risks of jogging. Although some were rightly critical of previously sedentary, overweight individuals beginning a jogging program without medical supervision, a vocal minority adamantly argued that running was dangerous for healthy adults as well and might even be fatal. A widely publicized 1976 article in *Playboy*, illustrated with a jogging skeleton, claimed that "running or jogging is one of the most wasteful and hazardous forms of exercise." According to physician J. E. Schmidt, jogging caused prematurely drooping breasts and herniated spinal disks, among other maladies, and it unnecessarily jostled the heart.[129] Physician Peter Steincrohn continued his campaign against vigorous exercise with a new book that warned about the hazards of jogging. In *How to Cure Your Jog-germania*, Steincrohn related stories of joggers who had suddenly dropped dead while running and cited studies that had found no correlation between exercise and health. He cautioned, "If you're pushing 40 that's exercise enough." Steincrohn argued that fitness could be achieved through diet, smoking avoidance, alcohol moderation, breathing exercises, and lifestyle changes designed to reduce stress.[130] The 1980 book *Jogging: The Dance of Death*—which claimed that, under the right conditions, jogging could kill almost anyone, even those without a history of heart disease—is evidence that uncertainty about the benefits of exercise lasted into the next decade.[131]

The argument against jogging was strengthened by numerous anecdotal reports of sudden death occurring during or shortly after a run.[132] By 1984, when Jim Fixx died during an afternoon run, the running community had formulated a ready response to critics who charged that running was dangerous: Runners such as Fixx had dramatically improved their health through their exercise routines, rectifying much of the damage done to their bodies by smoking, a sedentary lifestyle, and an unhealthy diet. A running habit, proponents argued, extended the lives of these people, and Fixx and others like him would have died much earlier if they had not been runners.[133] Interestingly, for many joggers, a death like Fixx's was a desirable end to life. Running literature was peppered with references to death, and joggers often wrote that they hoped to expire on the trail rather than endure a slow, painful decline. Few observers saw the irony that sudden death from a heart attack—the midcentury problem jogging had been invented to remedy—was now seen as the best way to go.[134]

Part of the difficulty of making sense of the medical advice aimed at joggers was the diversity of the jogging public. Whereas a significant segment of the running population engaged in modest jogging for cardiovascular health, a growing proportion had extended their runs substantially. Discussion about health risks seemed to intensify as many joggers abandoned exercise routines designed to improve health and embraced long-distance running as a measure of accomplishment and a demonstration of self-mastery. Thomas J. Bassler, founder of the American Medical Joggers Association (a group of running health professionals affiliated with the National Jogging Association), was a tireless promoter who claimed that regular marathon running provided total protection from heart attacks.[135] Bassler, a pathologist by training, reviewed autopsy reports and conducted his own postmortem examinations of marathon runners, determining that none had died of coronary heart disease.[136] Bassler claimed that jogging short distances, such as those recommended by Cooper, Bowerman, and Harris, produced no beneficial effects and that regular runs of at least six miles were necessary for heart health.[137] He went so far as to correlate specific distances with the duration of protection, claiming that one marathon finished in four to six hours earned six years of protection from coronary heart disease.[138] Despite skepticism by the medical establishment, Bassler's enthusiastic pronouncements continued until 1979, when four autopsied marathoners were found to have coronary atherosclerosis.[139] Bassler received much media attention throughout the decade, and although he served as a counter to equally vocal antijogging physicians, the extreme claims of both sides ultimately created confusion for the exercising health consumer.

Illustrating the uncertainty of many joggers, a 1979 U.S. News & World Report feature ran side-by-side interviews with pro and con physicians so readers could form their own opinions. Dr. Meyer Friedman, an antijogging cardiologist and developer of the type A–type B personality scheme, vigorously discouraged running, which had resulted in "hundreds of deaths." According to Friedman, running worsened coronary disease and raised blood pressure by causing a runner's heart to beat more vigorously. "There are no really lasting health benefits whatsoever from jogging," he argued. "So many people today are actually risking their lives by jogging." Alongside Friedman's interview, runner Dr. David Brody told readers that jogging lowered blood pressure and pulse rate and improved the heart's stroke volume. Although Brody conceded that insufficient statistical evidence had been collected to make a conclusive determination about jogging's benefits, he was unwilling to wait thirty years to learn the results of ongoing research.[140] Thus, like Brody, joggers plodded along, putting their faith in smaller studies showing that exercise lowered cholesterol levels and blood pressure, and hoping that these indicators of good health would ultimately lead to the unequivocal scientific validation of their efforts.

Even as jogging was repurposed into environmental symbiosis, spiritual practice, and self-help, interest in jogging for health reasons continued to grow, in spite of the ongoing debate over its benefits. The economic troubles of the 1970s exacerbated an already difficult climate for health care in the United States. Technological advances in medicine had led to higher costs that strained household budgets and government coffers; physicians were no longer perceived as having their patients' best interests at heart, and Americans began to question whether medical progress was entirely beneficial.[141] This decline in public confidence forced Americans to reconsider their relationships with their own bodies. Fed up with an increasingly unresponsive health care system, people became more interested in traditional healing and alternative health care; holistic medicine received more attention as health seekers looked beyond allopathic medicine to chiropody, osteopathy, and acupuncture. The establishment of community health care clinics, a renewed interest in home births and midwifery, and the publication of the Boston Women's Health Collective's *Our Bodies, Ourselves* were all part of this movement.[142] To second-generation joggers, running was another of these nontraditional therapies. Many joggers, for example, refused to see traditional physicians or doctors who did not jog themselves, believing that their bodies were fundamentally different from those of nonexercisers. Running cardiologist George Sheehan was one of the most vocal critics, arguing that doctors were only able to treat disease, not promote health.[143]

At the same time that running was imagined as a form of nontraditional medicine, it was understood by another cohort as a decidedly mainstream, even conservative, activity. Knowledge of disease risk factors had been mounting steadily over the previous two decades, creating the perception that health was entirely in the hands of the individual. This belief was also embraced by the federal government, which promoted preventive measures as a way to cut health care expenses. The surgeon general's 1979 report on health promotion and disease prevention, *Healthy People*, was the culmination of a decade of efforts that held the individual accountable for his or her lifestyle choices. In the report, Joseph Califano, secretary of the Department of Health, Education, and Welfare, admonished the nation, "We are killing ourselves by our own careless habits." Califano reminded Americans that "indulgences in 'private' excesses have results that are far from private," and he stated that "you, the individual, can do more for your own health and well-being than any doctor, any hospital, any drug, any exotic medical device."[144] This view of health promoted the idea that indiscriminate germs and random cell mutations played no role in illness: if you got sick, it was your own fault. Exercise, of course, was a crucial part of this philosophy. Jogging, according to Richard Bohannon, was a "do-it-yourself health-maintenance program."[145] The goal of his National Jogging Association "was to raise the consciousness of the American people; to get them to take personal responsibility for the fact that most diseases we die of are voluntary conditions."[146] Such rhetoric resonated with fiscally conservative politicians and citizens as both the nation and the field of medicine faced serious financial crises during the 1970s.

The crowd assembled for the inauguration of National Jogging Day, described at the beginning of this chapter, was representative of those who saw jogging as a money saver. When they took to the streets, they were visibly demonstrating concern for their own health as well as the nation's purse and their neighbors' tax dollars. When Stewart Udall opened four jogging trails in the Washington, D.C., area, he was accompanied by many members of Congress.[147] The running exploits of Senators William Proxmire (R-Wis.) and Richard Lugar (R-Ind.) were often cited as admirable models for fellow citizens. Proxmire wrote two consumer health guides, and Lugar often took part in National Jogging Day celebrations and praised the cost-saving efforts of joggers. "Individuals making free choices are saving the country millions of dollars annually by reducing demands on our health care facilities," he told the *Jogger* in 1978.[148]

Private industry also began to make a distinction between exercisers and nonexercisers. Occidental Life of North Carolina began to offer discounted insurance policies to serious runners (which it defined as those who ran at least three times a week for twenty minutes per session) in the

1970s. The company's regular ads in *Runner's World*, which depicted a trim man in running clothes supporting an overweight smoker on his shoulders, argued that fit people should not have to pay the same life insurance rates as the "static majority."[149] Edward Ayres, editor of the *Runner*, linked running with health care savings when he blamed nonexercisers for increased costs. "The people who give themselves heart attacks by refusing to perform even the most minimal maintenance on their bodies are the ones who drive up the cost of health care and insurance for the runner," he argued.[150] The result of such a philosophy—one that remains embedded in contemporary fitness culture—was to legitimize joggers' feelings of moral superiority. It also engendered further animosity between joggers and nonjoggers. Even more troubling was its foundation on the false notion that all Americans had equal access to fitness opportunities and health information, when it was clear that health promotion efforts were making only modest inroads in less affluent communities.

In the late 1960s and throughout the 1970s, millions of middle-class Americans regularly took to high school tracks, park trails, and their neighborhoods to combat heart disease, lower cholesterol, and ward off diseases linked to chronic inactivity. Jogging became popular because it channeled interest in exercise that had been building for almost twenty years into a specific activity that could be done almost anywhere by anyone. The easygoing, participatory nature of jogging attracted Americans who were new to exercise and were heeding warnings about the need for physical activity in everyday life. A second, younger generation of joggers joined this trend and used it as a way to demonstrate solidarity with political concerns. In its ability to unite joggers of all ages and political persuasions, jogging was truly the first form of exercise to become a mass movement. Unfortunately, joggers began to draw a line between those who had the time, money, and inclination to exercise and those who did not. In the next decade, this division would solidify, creating a new meritocracy of the fit body that was determined not only by mileage but also by musculature.

Jogging brought healthy living to the cultural forefront. While earlier national discussions of fitness had brought attention to the idea of exercise, they had not provided the means to take action. The origins of the jogging movement have not been well documented. Too often, jogging's roots in health promotion have been obscured in favor of a narrative that views the new phenomenon with bemusement or even derision. Its success is a testimony to the effectiveness of public health campaigns, but it also speaks to their limitations. Preventive health messages did not permeate all levels of society equally, as disparate jogging participation rates make clear. In its normalization, jogging became more widely available but also more exclusive. Race entrance fees, pricey running shoes and clothing, training manuals, and lack of knowledge constituted barriers to widespread participation. Even as it functioned as a critique of the affluent lifestyle it was supposed to remedy, jogging was quickly and enthusiastically absorbed by a consumer culture that appropriated it for profit.

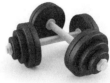

5

In 1979, President Jimmy Carter collapsed during a
10-kilometer (6.2-mile) run at Camp David. Because the
race was a staged media event, numerous journalists and
photographers were on hand to witness the president fall to
his knees near the 4-mile mark. Colman McCarthy, a regular runner and syndicated columnist, reported that Carter's
"legs wobbled, his face drained of color and he sagged help-
lessly into the arms of two aides."[1] Photos of the stumbling
Carter appeared in newspapers and magazines across the
country.[2] Carter's inability to complete the race seemed to
reflect his political difficulties. Many could not help but
draw comparisons between Carter's collapse and charges of
weak and ineffective leadership. "Is this the kind of man—
so blindly determined that he is unwilling to discontinue
a foolhardy enterprise for which he is unprepared—that
we want running the country?" one letter writer queried
the *Washington Post*.[3] McCarthy cast doubt on Carter's pur-
ported running regimen, wondering why a man who had
completed the course four times previously and claimed
to have clocked a 6:30 mile would be unable to finish the
race.[4] Many viewed the Camp David event as an attempt to
highlight Carter's physical vigor and a political maneuver to
suggest that opponent Ronald Reagan's age made him unfit
for the presidency. Nearly a year later, as the campaign grew
more heated, Carter's failure to finish still plagued him.

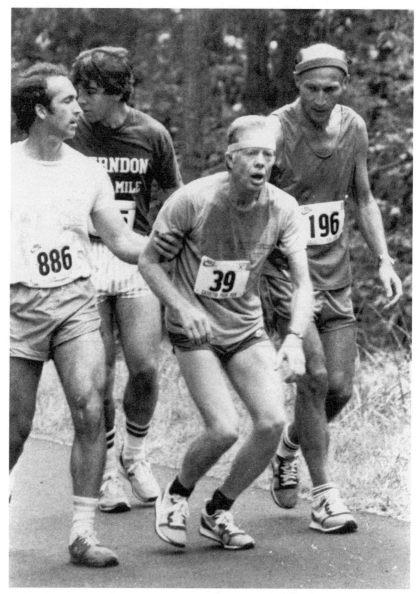

By the mid-1970s, jogging had become a way to demonstrate personal competency and success. In 1979, President Jimmy Carter took part in a ten-kilometer run at Camp David to highlight his physical vigor and suggest that challenger Ronald Reagan was too old to hold the presidency. Carter's failure to complete the race would dog him for the remainder of his term. (© Phil Stewart)

Journalist Mark Shields advised Carter to give up his hobby, charging that "jogging is not presidential. . . . Jogging does not simply remind voters that you are younger than Reagan; it reminds them of that day of the Camp David Marathon."[5]

Four years later, a seventy-two-year-old Ronald Reagan successfully mobilized popular interest in physical fitness for political gain. In 1983, Reagan appeared on the cover of *Parade* magazine (a Sunday supplement to many American newspapers) wearing a white T-shirt and doing biceps curls on a Nautilus machine. The photo was part of a cover story, authored by Reagan, that detailed his physical fitness program. One caption stated that the president's chest measurement had increased by nearly two inches since beginning a weight-training regimen after surviving a 1981 assassination attempt. A 1941 Hollywood publicity photo of the toned actor in swim trunks showed Reagan's enviable physique in his younger years. The article demonstrated Reagan's awareness of modern fitness trends while also invoking a specifically American ruggedness in describing his current conditioning program. His strength training routine at the White House employed free weights and Nautilus machines, while time spent at his California ranch included traditional farm chores ("pumping firewood") and horseback riding.[6]

Reagan and his advisers smartly capitalized on the relatively new association between physical vitality and professional capability. The *Parade* article made it clear that Reagan was healthy, youthful, and active, while at the same time implying that the president's exercise program enhanced not only his physical strength but also his ability to govern. Even if Carter had been able to finish his race, running didn't convey the same message that weight lifting did. Reagan and his team demonstrated their awareness that fitness had been redefined: in the 1980s, sculpted muscles were the goal.

Exercise in the new decade was marked by a turn away from the health concerns that had preoccupied Americans in earlier years. There was a new interest in shaping the body's outward appearance. Health concerns didn't vanish entirely, but now the idea that exercise resulted in better health seemed to be a foregone conclusion.[7] In earlier decades, much of exercise culture had centered on the process of exercise—that is, the act of

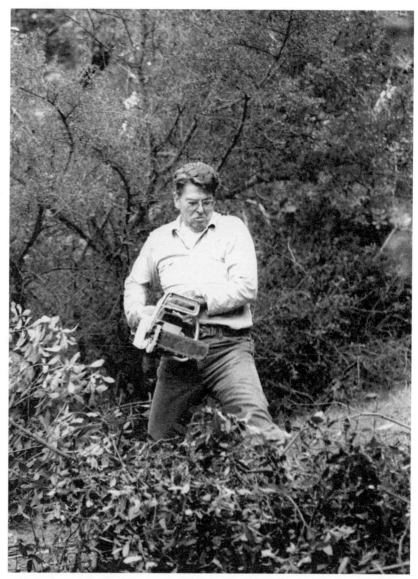

The 1980s was the decade of the "power physique," when muscles became a symbol of the new national toughness. President Ronald Reagan demonstrated his awareness of both old and new notions of fitness on his California ranch, where he cleared brush and "pumped firewood," and in Washington, where he frequently mentioned his weight-lifting routine. In the photo on the right, Reagan is standing next to NFL coach George Allen, chair of the President's Council on Physical Fitness and Sports. (Ronald Reagan Library)

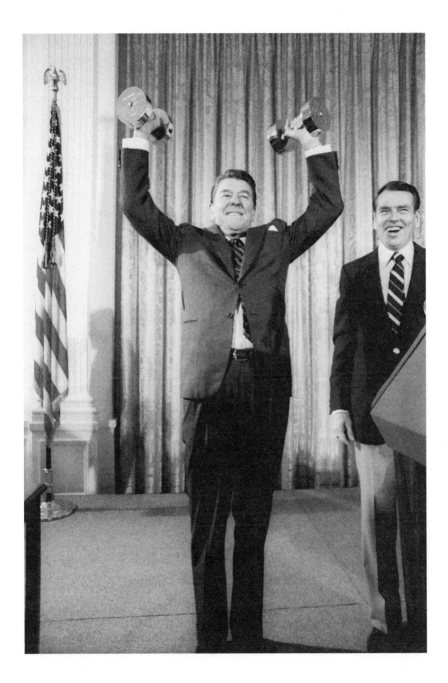

becoming healthy. In the 1980s, exercise culture became much more focused on the result. As one weight-lifting equipment manufacturer put it, "People are saying 'To hell with the heart and lungs and all this marathon running stuff—I want to look better, not like somebody who just got out of a prisoner-of-war camp.'"[8]

The new focus on muscles meant that fitness moved from the track to the gym.[9] By the 1980s, commercial health clubs had been promoting their services for roughly three decades, and 7 million Americans were spending $5 billion each year on membership fees.[10] Health clubs were not an invention of the 1980s, but the decade's emphasis on aesthetics gave new importance to shaping the body and displaying the effects of a workout long after one had left the gym. As Nicolaus Mills wrote, "The 1980s were not only the decade of the power lunch and the power tie, but the power physique."[11] The muscular physique was an apt symbol for a nation led by a president who made no apologies for his militaristic policies. Ronald Reagan and the culture of victory espoused by his presidency were reflected in a new toughness in Americans' personal exercise regimens. As one fitness instructor pointed out, "People want a more rigorous exercise program than they used to. Things used to be nirvana-oriented—getting to know yourself, meditation. But it's a tougher world today than in the 60s or 70s and people want to toughen up to fight back."[12] Paradoxically, even as weight-lifting aficionados pumped more, exercised longer, and sought to outdo the member on the next bench, health clubs became a new kind of community center for many Americans.

THE GENTRIFICATION OF THE GYM

The idea of a dedicated space for the maintenance of the body has existed since at least the 1830s in the United States.[13] Around the turn of the century, private athletic clubs offered upper-class men, and occasionally women, a refined environment for socialization, entertainment, and physical development. These members-only clubs played an important role in the popularization of physical conditioning as a leisure pastime in the early twentieth century. Club athletic facilities typically included a gymnasium with weights, pulleys, and Indian clubs; racquetball and squash courts; a swimming pool; and, space permitting, a running track. The maintenance of such a wide array of facilities was costly; athletic clubs were difficult ventures to manage, even in times of economic prosperity. Beginning in the 1920s, athletic clubs suffered a number of financial setbacks that drastically decreased their numbers and, at the same time, eroded the belief that physical culture was an appropriate hobby for upstanding men. The enactment of Prohibition ended the lucrative in-house sales of alcohol that had kept many clubs solvent. Membership rosters thinned with the Depression, wartime deployment, and competition from suburban country clubs. As a result, athletic clubs declined and eventually disappeared from most American cities.[14] By the time of the men's cardiac crisis in the 1950s, bodybuilding and weight lifting—activities specifically associated with the gym—were regarded as unrefined. The gym space itself was imagined as dark, dank, and somewhat louche.

By midcentury, however, a number of trends coalesced to rehabilitate the perception of exercise in general and of the gym in particular. Beginning in the 1950s, health club entrepreneurs reimagined the gym as a place of luxury and constructed facilities with elaborate décor, bright lighting, and a club atmosphere. At the same time, workplace fitness initiatives changed the perception of *who* engaged in exercise. The cardiac crisis and physician endorsement began to legitimate physical conditioning for men. Workplace gyms made it convenient to exercise and injected a sense of virtue into exercising by associating it with employment. These two trends coincided with the expansion of exercise within the beauty industry; reducing salons and day spas ensconced women's fitness in an upscale environment that made toning and weight reduction seem less of a chore and more of a luxury. Together, these influences gentrified the gym and normalized the practice of exercise. According to one *Newsweek* estimate, 5 million Americans frequented reducing salons and gymnasiums in 1959, evidence that dedicated exercise was becoming increasingly popular.[15] That gyms were used as the setting for several episodes of popular midcentury television shows, including *Tightrope*, *The Bob Cummings Show*, *The Jack Benny Show*, and *The Green Hornet*, also demonstrates their growing cultural acceptance.[16]

Clubs that catered to a middle-class clientele invoked a sense of luxury and refinement through their physical surroundings. Proprietors hoped this feeling of opulence would link their establishments to older notions of athletic clubs, country clubs, and the few independent clubs that catered to the ultrawealthy.[17] At the same time, this need to provide a certain physical environment highlights the considerable resistance health promoters faced in convincing Americans to exercise. Former bodybuilder Vic Tanny's eponymous chain was the first and best known of the new middle-class health clubs. Believing that "good health can be merchandized just like automobiles," Tanny helped transform the nascent fitness industry through his aggressive marketing and his luxury facilities that were designed to appeal to both sexes. The business depended on a fast-growing clientele, which was developed nearly exclusively through television advertising. Tanny spent $2 million annually on commercials that promoted the chain's "family atmosphere," while encouraging prospective members to "take it off, build it up, make it firm." By 1959, Tanny clubs had about half a million members.[18]

Inspired by the memory of the first gym he had ever visited, which "smelled like a locker room and . . . was so dark I could barely see my own muscles," Tanny transformed the gym into a glitzy, gilded, spa-like environment; exercise equipment was chrome plated to make members feel as if they had come to "treat themselves," not to work.[19] All the Tanny gyms featured swimming pools, steam baths, massage rooms, and sun rooms. One West Hempstead, New York, location even had a movie theater, two bowling alleys, and a skating rink with pink ice, all free of charge for members.[20] Specifications for new Tanny gyms in the New York area required 10,000 square feet of space and a swimming pool or the possibility to build one.[21] Newsweek described the clubs as "glittering, cocktail-lounge modern sweat parlors," and a writer for the Saturday Evening Post dubbed the style "Miami Flamboyant." Apparently, not all the clubs measured up to the Long Island location, though. A visitor to one of Tanny's busiest New York City clubs described it as having "all the charm of a tool foundry."[22]

A second major chain of the era was Ray Wilson and Bob Delmonteque's American Health Studios (AHS), which opened in the early 1950s and expanded to more than 300 properties before folding in 1959 because of financial problems. Their gyms, "luxuriously decorated in chrome, mirrors, carpeting [and] leatherette," included weights, sauna, pool, and

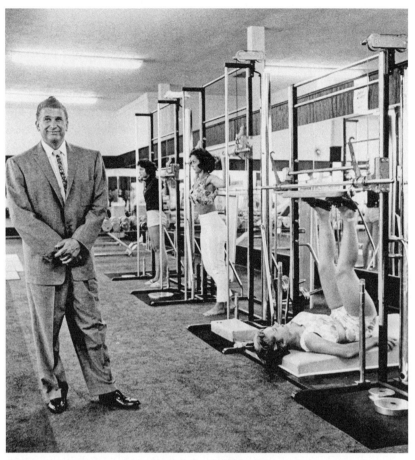

Entrepreneur Vic Tanny nearly single-handedly rehabilitated the popular perception of gyms by redesigning their interiors to suggest luxury and refinement through the use of carpeting, mirrors, and chrome. Tanny's chain expanded to eighty-eight locations before becoming insolvent. This photo was likely taken on a "ladies' day"—before the mid-1970s, men and women typically alternated days at commercial health clubs. (Photograph by Allan Grant, Time & Life Pictures, Getty Images)

steam baths in air-conditioned facilities that "flavored exercise and made it taste good."[23] Delmonteque and Wilson relied heavily on newspaper advertising to attract members, and they cast a wide net in terms of clientele. One ad specifically addressed businessmen—asking, "Desk Fatigue?"— and promoted exercise's ability to increase circulation and mental alertness. Other ads that appealed to male vanity had more in common with the working-class body ideal popularized by Charles Atlas. Featuring the image of a well-sculpted bodybuilder (possibly Delmonteque himself), one *Los Angeles Times* ad told readers they could "be the man of her ideals."[24] AHS ads often promoted reduced fees for "advanced bodybuilders" ($1 per month, in comparison to regular fees ranging from $3 to $5), undoubtedly hoping to attract a cohort of muscular members whose bodies would testify to the effectiveness of the club's program. While this dual middle-class/working-class appeal was somewhat unusual, it reflected the increasing prominence of the muscular physique in Hollywood.[25]

Reducing salons (also called figure salons) and day spas represented another important segment of the growing fitness market. The arrival of exercise classes in spas and salons attested to the intense weight-consciousness of the 1960s and illustrated that exercise for women was seen as a beauty treatment. Revenue derived from weight reduction and figure control in the cosmetology industry was negligible in 1957, but just five years later, it totaled $30 million.[26] Elizabeth Arden salons had long advocated exercise to improve posture and develop poise. In New York, instructor Marjorie Craig directed the program where she had taught toning classes since 1952.[27] Massages were a particular specialty of the beauty industry. The physical manipulation of surplus avoirdupois was believed to help flush fat out of the system. In Elizabeth Arden's Washington, D.C., location, four European-trained masseuses were on hand to rub excess flesh into submission at $6 an hour. It was also possible to avail oneself of the "shake away" chair, the steam cabinet (heavy perspiration was thought to aid weight loss), and private exercise instruction.[28] Helena Rubenstein salons offered "beauty stretch" classes, which employed a pink rubber cable similar to Jack La Lanne's Glamour-Stretcher, in addition to massage, electrical stimulation, a dry heat cabinet, and diet analysis.[29] Typically featuring all-female staffs, spas and reducing salons also provided women an entrée into the burgeoning fitness industry.[30]

Slenderella, established in 1946, was the best known of the three most popular reducing salon chains of the era (the others were Stauffer and Silhouette). Although reducing salons were not health clubs per se, they helped entrench the habit of visiting a location outside the home for the

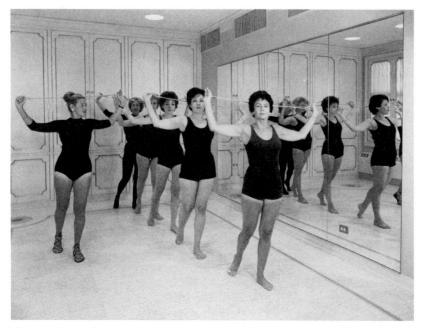

The cosmetology industry was a major source of fitness information for women in the 1950s and 1960s. Because women's exercise was considered a beauty practice, spas and salons routinely offered fitness instruction. In this 1962 image, women at the Helena Rubenstein salon in New York develop their posture. (Photograph by Samuel H. Gottscho, Gottscho-Schleisner Collection, Prints and Photographs Division, Library of Congress, LC G613-77413-A)

improvement of one's body. These establishments specialized in passive or so-called effortless exercise: the client sat or reclined on a device that vibrated or rolled the flesh, on the premise that, like massage, manipulation of fat could speed its breakdown. Figure salons appealed to women who wanted to shape their bodies but found exercise distasteful, perhaps because they believed that vigorous physical activity was not feminine. The popularity of these devices made them a fixture in many gyms frequented by men as well; some machines, such as the Stauffer System magic couch, were available for retail sale as well.[31]

With European "princesses" for spokesmodels, the Slenderella chain marketed an image of glamour, reportedly serving 3 million clients in 110 locations by 1956.[32] During a typical visit—which the chain claimed was the equivalent of riding ten miles on horseback or playing thirty-six holes

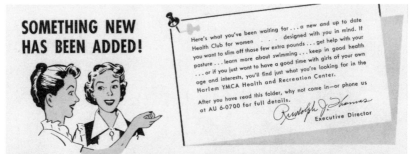

SOMETHING NEW HAS BEEN ADDED!

Here's what you've been waiting for . . . a new and up to date Health Club for women . . . designed with you in mind. If you want to slim off those few extra pounds . . . get help with your posture . . . learn more about swimming . . . keep in good health . . . or if you just want to have a good time with girls of your own age and interests, you'll find just what you're looking for in the Harlem YMCA Health and Recreation Center.

After you have read this folder, why not come in—or phone us at AU 6-0700 for full details.

Rudolph J. Thomas
Executive Director

AN UP TO DATE WOMAN'S DEPARTMENT AT HARLEM BRANCH YMCA

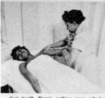

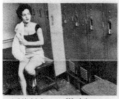

Feel tired? There's nothing more relaxing after a hard day than a good, soothing massage. Licensed masseuse is on duty.

Individual lockers . . . 500 of them . . . for members of the new center. Everything planned for YOUR privacy and convenience.

FOR THE BODY BEAUTIFUL

Complete Physical Education Program
Fully Equipped Gymnasium
Swimming Pool
Individual and Group Sports

Massage	Heat Cabinet
Rest Cots	Sun Lamp
Showers	Conditioning Classes

Masseuse on Duty

FOR YOUR ENJOYMENT

Complete Social Program
Television Lounge
Restaurant
Parties
Social Dancing
Tennis
Volleyball
Basketball

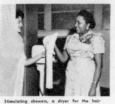

Stimulating showers, a dryer for the hair . . . all equipment bought with YOU in mind . . . to help you look your best.

A COMPLETE PROGRAM FOR WOMEN OF ALL AGES

The Health and Recreation Center is the most recent development in the Harlem YMCA's program of service to its community. The items listed above are only a few of the many features which are now being offered to women of all ages.

The area occupied by the center has been specially equipped and decorated to meet the needs of women members. Every care has been taken to provide the utmost in pleasant surroundings, comfort and convenience.

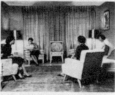

The television lounge of the new department is modern and attractive . . . truly designed for milady's comfort.

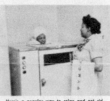

Here's a popular way to relax and get rid of a few extra pounds at the same time . . . Plan to enjoy our up-to-date heat cabinet.

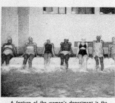

A feature of the women's department is the swimming program. Expert instruction is available for those who want or need it.

This brochure for the Woman's Department at the Harlem YMCA is similar to promotional pamphlets for the YMCA's Business Men's Clubs. BMC advertising often highlighted nap rooms and relaxation facilities rather than exercise opportunities. BMCs were generally not open to women; that the Harlem location admitted women speaks to the racially segregated nature of the reducing salons and spas that middle-class women frequented for exercise. (Kautz Family YMCA Archives) of golf—clients were instructed to lie back on padded, vibrating massage tables, fully clothed but with bra unhooked and girdle removed.[33] Sessions usually lasted forty-five minutes, and clients listened to music while they slenderized.[34] The fee was $2 per appointment, although sessions were usually sold in packages ranging from $60 to $350.[35] Slenderella also offered customized meal plans, a line of dietetic foods, and a girdle called "Magic Skin."[36] The almost too-good-to-be-true advertisements boasted a weight-loss system that employed "no harmful drugs, no massages, no exercises, no electricity, no steam baths, no undressing, no strict dieting."[37]

The success of Slenderella and its competitors might be attributable more to participation in some type of program than to the doubtful benefits of passive exercise. As one Washington, D.C., woman put it, "When [my husband] knows I'm paying for reducing sessions I HAVE to control my eating."[38] Another client ascribed salons' claims of success to their measuring techniques: on arrival, new customers were measured with a loose measuring tape; at the end of the treatment program, the tape was held taut.[39] Although methods such as massage, vibration, and passive exercise might seem laughable to modern exercisers, in the absence of a widespread understanding of exercise physiology, their appeal is understandable. This seems especially true given the limitless sense of technological progress that infused midcentury popular culture. Homes were filled with previously unimaginable appliances, and décor influences came from space travel.[40] If a man could travel to the moon and back, why couldn't a machine help one shed a few pounds?

Moreover, these passive methods were comparable to the activities many gym members engaged in at midcentury.[41] Before fitness was defined in cardiovascular terms, the benefits of going to the gym were just as likely to be derived from relaxation, a sense of caring for one's body, and socializing as from a vigorous exercise session. For men who frequented the YMCA's Business Men's Clubs (BMCs), exercise was only part of the club experience. A promotional brochure for the Rochester, New York, BMC highlighted the club's relaxation facilities to the near exclusion of its exercise equipment. Of the nine photographs used to entice new members, only one depicted any form of exercise—men on stationary bikes. The other eight photos illustrated relaxation and leisure in the hot room, massage room, lounge ("air-conditioned with radio and TV"), steam room, rest room, whirlpool bath, and ultraviolet "sunbaths."[42]

In 1958, *New York Times* writer Barney Lefferts calculated that New York City had approximately three dozen health clubs with 15,000 members paying about $150 annually. He estimated that there were four "ghost members"—those who came to the club to use the sunlamp, steam room, and massage facilities only—for every one person who came to exercise.[43] Although Lefferts admitted that many of the "non-athletic" members also did "'table work' consisting of leg-lifting and the like, for most," he observed, "the routine consisted of three minutes of ultra-violet light, twenty minutes relaxing on a deck chair in the hot room (160 degrees), steam bath for five, a hard-boiled egg for restoration and a shave." The exclusive ambience seemed to be the health club's most appealing feature. As one manager put it, "'Turkish' bath today is a dirty word to Three-Button Joe from Madison Avenue. But tell him it's the Swanky Dank Health and Conditioning Society and he'll join up."[44]

Through the 1960s and 1970s, the health club industry expanded rapidly, adding chains and independent gyms. A 1974 survey of Manhattan workout facilities showed that although fitness studios (emphasizing classes for which participants typically paid per session) were still plentiful, all-inclusive health clubs, "the newest trend in exercise palaces," were gaining in popularity.[45] Four years later, the *New York Times* noted that "hardly a neighborhood is without a club."[46]

WORKPLACE FITNESS

Commercial ventures such as figure salons and health clubs formed the foundation of the modern fitness industry. They rehabilitated the image of the gym and acquainted Americans with the idea of exercise in a designated space outside the home. The establishment of on-site exercise facilities at work similarly contributed to the upscaling of exercise. New company gyms were bright, modern facilities designed to inspire, but the fact that these gyms were employer sponsored changed the nature of exercise. Employees at company gyms were goal oriented; unlike the socializing described earlier by BMC habitués, executives who took part in company programs were there for a purpose—to ensure their fitness for work.

The presence of a fitness director or medical director meant that exercise was serious business. As workplace fitness programs became increasingly common, they contributed to the redefinition of exercise as labor intensive and, in tandem with the jogging movement, as necessarily strenuous. The association of a fit body and labor, both on the job and in the gym, injected a virtuous component into an exercise regimen.

American businesses first became interested in men's health in the 1950s, when the coronary crisis, described in detail in chapter 3, created fear that a large segment of the executive workforce was at risk of heart attack and death.[47] For those men who survived a heart attack, standard recovery prescriptions still meant a long absence from work—as long as six months in many cases.[48] In an era when a man typically worked at the same company for his entire career, the loss of a single employee entailed a serious loss of productivity and expertise. According to the American Heart Association, recruiting replacements for the 200,000 men between the ages of forty-five and sixty-five who were disabled or killed by heart disease cost businesses $700 million every year.[49] As a result, many companies began to offer physical examinations, nutrition education, and on-site exercise facilities. For middle-class men, the most influential source of health and fitness information in this era may have been the workplace.

Through the 1960s and 1970s, it became the norm to work out at work. The list of major corporations that installed on-site fitness facilities was long. Philips Petroleum, Goodyear, Texas Instruments, American Can Company, Kimberly-Clark, Chase Manhattan, Aetna, General Foods, Pepsi, Gates Rubber, Exxon, Xerox, Weyerhauser, and Atlas Van Lines were among those with extensive on-site fitness facilities.[50] Companies spared no expense in setting up elaborate, state-of-the-art fitness centers, making exercise a desired fringe benefit. Companies that couldn't offer on-site programs (usually because of space limitations) purchased corporate memberships at private facilities.[51] By 1974, work-site exercise programs had become such a trend that a membership association was formed for their directors, who numbered more than 500 four years later.[52] By 1980, more than 3,000 businesses offered health and fitness programs for employees.[53] The fitness trend in business was so significant that hotels catering to business travelers began to install workout facilities.[54]

Because being overweight was a risk factor for heart attacks, some firms also conducted nutrition education. International Telephone and Telegraph, the Port Authority of New York, and Chase Manhattan Bank were among the companies that listed calorie counts for meals served in employee dining rooms to increase nutritional awareness. Some even offered financial incentives to employees who lost weight or maintained an exercise regimen. For instance, Edward Lowe, president of Lowe's Inc., a Michigan-based manufacturer, formed the "I Can't Afford to Lose You Club." Under this program, managers stood to gain 1.5 percent of their salary for weight loss completed by and maintained after a target date.[55]

Vestiges of the cardiac crisis remained, in that most workplace wellness programs were limited to middle or upper management. Although studies had disproved the widely held notion that only hard-driving executives were heart attack prone, lower-level employees were typically excluded from wellness plans. For instance, Chase Manhattan's calorie-counting menus appeared only in its main and private dining rooms; the program did not extend to the cafeteria used by "lower-echelon" employees. These exclusionary policies were typically defended by the explanation that firms had greater financial investments in their senior employees, who, they claimed, tended to be older and subject to more stress than their junior colleagues.[56] The indirect effect of this practice, however, was to bestow an aura of exclusivity on working out, furthering the belief that exercise was a hobby of the well-to-do.

Media coverage of corporate fitness programs and the executives who participated in them gradually created a profile of the ideal professional as a man who was serious about both his work and his exercise routine. The hard-driving personality traits that were said to lead to success in business (and increased one's risk of a heart attack) were now expressed in one's fitness regimen. The portrait of a CEO who skipped lunch to run five miles or who left the office after a long day and spent seventy-five minutes exercising at the gym became typical in the popular press and business publications.[57] A 1968 *Newsweek* article noted that the presidents of Pepsi, Transamerica, Wells Fargo, and Pacific Gas and Electric, as well as the magazine's own president, had taken up jogging.[58] One Texas firm, the Tyler Corporation, even sponsored the Tyler Cup, a fitness competition for executives.[59] "The locker room is joining the board room as an integral part of corporate life," the New York Times noted in 1978.[60] One study found that by 1987, 91 percent of all executives exercised.[61]

Workplace exercise programs were so successful in rehabilitating the image of the exerciser that even the stereotype of the "dumb jock" was reversed. By the late 1970s, executives were expected to look like they were in shape. One personal trainer in Chicago attributed her growing number of male clients to the fact that a beer belly had become "the kiss of death to any man who wants to get ahead in business or professional life."[62] An employee who did not look fit was presumed to lack discipline and to be neither well organized nor high functioning. An industry analyst warned that "managers are getting reluctant to hire or promote individuals who show signs that they aren't in control of their health," and at least one study showed that the overweight earned less than their average-weight counterparts.[63] A fit body and the virtuous personality traits associated with it opened the door to weight discrimination in the workplace, based on the belief that overweight employees lacked the personal character-istics necessary for success in business. Business Week reported on "the fat personality" that inhibited go-getter traits. According to the head of Weight Watchers in Atlanta, the overweight "sit in the background and wait for promotions. They are bashful and ashamed to come forth because of their appearance."[64]

Workplace fitness programs continued to expand through the 1980s. The explosive growth of commercial health clubs increased their currency as fringe benefits, and firms became convinced of their effectiveness in increasing employee morale and physical wellness and decreasing ab-senteeism.[65] Workplace fitness initiatives played a crucial role in aligning the moral qualities considered desirable in the workplace with personal fitness routines. By the 1980s, the career-minded workforce had trans-formed exercise from a leisure hobby grounded in health to a statement of personal and professional competence written on the body.

THE MUSCULAR BODY

As noted in previous chapters, there is a long history of interaction be-tween the pursuit of bodybuilding and gay men. While the development of strength was often associated with masculinity, the cultivation of the body for its own sake was understood as less than masculine. The association between bodybuilding and homosexuality was concretely linked by the physique magazines of the 1950s and 1960s, which depicted straight bodybuilders posing, often knowingly, for gay readers. The homosocial atmosphere of the gym and the physical intimacy shared by bodybuilders also contributed to the widespread perception that many of them were gay. During the 1970s, the muscular physique was reclaimed as heterosexual, even as it grew in popularity among gay men; both groups popularized weight training and, consequently, the gym as the means to a shared physical ideal.[66]

The legitimation of visible musculature for straight men began in the mid-1970s with the growing fame of an Austrian bodybuilder named Arnold Schwarzenegger. Schwarzenegger, who had already made one Hollywood film, was the subject of *Pumping Iron*, a 1974 book written by Charles Gaines and photographed by George Butler, as well as a 1977 documentary of the same name.[67] The film followed Schwarzenegger and a group of competitors (including Lou Ferrigno, later of TV *Hulk* fame) as they prepared for the 1975 Mr. Olympia and Mr. Universe competitions. It was clear even before the film's release that interest in physical culture was growing. To raise funds to make the documentary, codirector George Butler staged a bodybuilding exhibition featuring Schwarzenegger at New York's Whitney Museum in 1976. In spite of a raging blizzard, more than five thousand people attended "The Art of Bodybuilding," which opened with a panel discussion among several art critics on the body in art, followed by a posing session. Expecting only a few hundred spectators, Butler was astounded at the show's turnout, and the cash drawer at the admission booth quickly filled. "We took in so much money we had to put it in piles on the floor," Butler later recalled.[68]

At the same time that *Pumping Iron* was engendering interest in bodybuilding, gay men were popularizing a more muscular appearance. The gay liberation movement helped dispel pervasive stereotypes of gay men as thin, pale, and limp-wristed. In the years after Stonewall, gay men asserted that they were men in full, not deviant "sissies." This affirmation of masculinity led to the development of a style of cultural presentation that took archetypal masculine figures and reinterpreted them for a gay lifestyle. "Clones," as they were known, adopted styles of dress rooted in blue-collar masculinity, such as the woodsman, cowboy, and construction worker. As one twenty-one-year-old described the scene in 1974, "Everyone looked like the Marlboro Man."[69] Clone style also called for a gym-built body, which contributed an even greater sense of masculinity to the already manly apparel. As one gym-goer explained to an interviewer, "Society sees musclemen as more masculine so I work out putting in long hours in the gym pumping iron. The results make me feel butch."[70]

As the predominant style of self-presentation among gay men in the 1970s, the clone was overtly sexual. At a casual glance, clone clothing resembled garments worn by straight men, but subtle clues informed knowledgeable onlookers of the wearer's sexuality. Clones' clothing fit closer to the body, and their grooming was more fastidious. Men often drew attention to the crotch by bleaching the fabric of their jeans or leaving the top button unfastened.[71] Designer Calvin Klein, whose first clothing collection was inspired by clone culture, continued this trend, popularizing the new erotic sensibility in men's fashion. In Klein's underwear line and in his suggestive marketing campaigns, which featured young, hairless models and athletes, the new vogue in muscular physiques turned men's bodies into objects of desire.[72] Clone culture was part of a larger trend during the late 1970s and early 1980s that sexualized the male body. Middle-class men's bodies underwent a process of aestheticization, much like the transformation of working-class men's bodies in the 1920s and 1930s.[73] Fitness culture and clone culture, aided by the new 1970s singles scene, raised appearance standards for gay and straight men alike.

Clone culture reconfirmed the long association between bodybuilding and gay men. When Butler was looking for a publisher for *Pumping Iron*, one prospective publishing house told him that "no one in America will buy a book of pictures of these half-clothed men of dubious sexual pursuits."[74] At the same time, however, Schwarzenegger and the *Pumping Iron* franchise claimed bodybuilding as the province of straight men. In scenes from the film, Schwarzenegger and his cohorts were shown with girlfriends and families. In the book, he was photographed carrying a topless woman on his shoulders, and other bodybuilders made mention of their

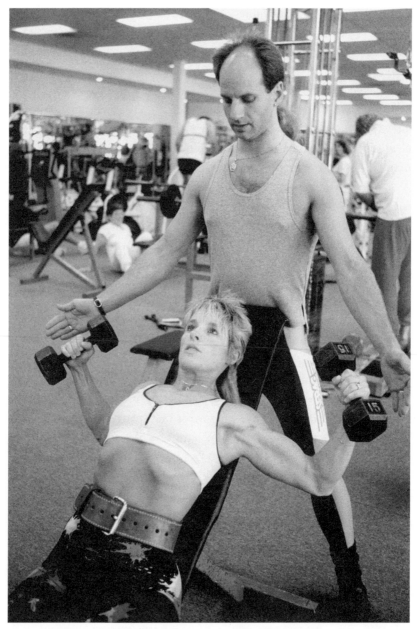

The pursuit of muscle for both men and women represented a new aesthetic turn in fitness culture. The prohibitive cost of weight training equipment made gym membership a necessity. After jogging, weight lifting was the nation's most popular recreational sport during the 1980s. (© Karl Weatherly/Corbis)

wives.[75] His movie roles similarly illustrated that a muscular physique was not necessarily a gay one. Schwarzenegger nearly single-handedly legitimated straight men's interest in bodybuilding. As one Schwarzenegger profile explained, "Before *Pumping Iron*, musclemen were weird, too masculine in their hulking forms, too feminine in their sideshow vanity."[76]

What the gay gym crowd and the world of serious bodybuilding had in common was a shared *disinterest* in the health benefits of working out. For both, aesthetics were the motivating force. Clones frequented a social circuit that included gyms, bars, nightclubs, and discos.[77] The pervasive use of recreational drugs by gay men who frequented the club scene illustrated that health concerns took second place to appearance.[78] As gay amateur bodybuilder Lenny Giteck joked, "Why have I engaged in all that huffing and puffing? For the health benefits . . . and if you believe *that*, there's a Florida swamp I can get you a great deal on."[79] Similarly, professional bodybuilders, who were judged in competitions by their physical symmetry and proportion, regularly sacrificed their health for the sake of competition-worthy physiques. In the weeks preceding a meet, they regularly followed strict diets designed to radically decrease body fat and increase the visibility of muscle mass. In the days preceding a competition, some men might not drink anything (even water), for fear of obscuring muscle striation beneath the skin. Outside of competitions, they consumed large amounts of protein powder and other natural and synthetic supplements designed to increase muscle mass.[80] Finally, the use of steroids was endemic. According to Gaines, most bodybuilders believed "that to stay competitive they have to use them."[81]

Clone style, in combination with the growing popularity of competitive bodybuilding and the fame of Arnold Schwarzenegger, had a tremendous influence on normative body shapes for both men and women, straight and gay. In 1980, the *New York Times* proclaimed, "This is the year to show your muscle."[82] That this ideal spread so rapidly in popular culture was due to changes in exercise technology that allowed novice gym-goers to strength-train with little knowledge or experience. Nautilus machines, invented by Florida weight-lifting enthusiast Arthur Jones, had become popular in the 1970s.[83] (The name of the equipment was derived from the shell-shaped cams that maintain constant resistance throughout an exercise.) Whereas free weights and cable equipment required a lifter to be familiar with the range of exercises for a given apparatus, Nautilus equipment was designed to work just one or two muscle groups per machine, required only a few mechanical adjustments by the exerciser, and often featured an instructional diagram. This new user-friendly equipment made the muscular ideal more attainable for novices. However, its prohibitive cost—in 1978, a full set of fourteen stations was $20,000 to $30,000—put it out of the price range of most home exercisers and made gym membership a necessity.[84] By the 1980s, weight lifting had become the second most popular recreational sport in America, after jogging.[85]

FITNESS CULTURE IN THE 1980S

The gentrification of the gym, the association of virtuous qualities with exercise, the popularization of the muscular physique, and the political zeitgeist came together to make the 1980s *the* fitness decade. Historians and casual observers of the fitness movement have termed the surge of interest in exercise during the 1980s a "boom," but as the previous chapters demonstrate, health experts and exercise entrepreneurs had been steadily promoting fitness as a life-saving measure, an appearance improver, and a leisure pastime for thirty years. An estimated 10.5 million Americans belonged to health clubs by 1988.[86] Even Americans who didn't take part in the exercise movement dressed as if they did—sneakers, track suits, leg warmers, and sweatbands were increasingly worn as fashion items rather than workout gear. Children couldn't escape fitness culture either: Mattel produced a Barbie doll that came with her own workout center, complete with a stationary bike and weights.[87]

Exercise culture was seemingly everywhere—in the gym, on the streets, and in popular culture at large. Motion pictures both implicitly and explicitly referenced exercise culture and the gym in particular. *Perfect* (1985), *Personal Best* (1982), *The Toxic Avenger* (1985), *On the Edge* (1985), and *Body and Soul* (1981) were all set in gyms and depicted characters whose lives were centered on fitness. Made-for-TV movies such as *Getting Physical* (1984) depicted the physical transformation of serious weight lifters. Popular music also reflected fitness trends. Olivia Newton John's "(Let's Get) Physical" (1982), as well as Diana Ross's "Muscles" (1982) and "Work that Body"

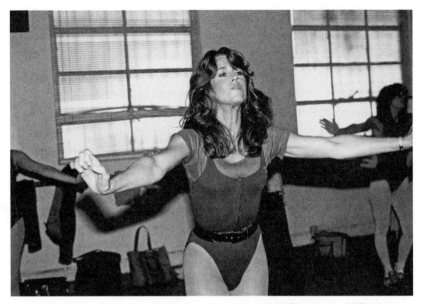

Jane Fonda was one of a number of celebrities who popularized the fitness-centered lifestyle. Her books and videos focused attention on aerobics and brought unprecedented numbers of women into the gym, fueling the expansion of the health club industry. In 1986, 90 percent of the nation's 24 million aerobic dancers were women. (© Bettman/Corbis)

(1982), were evidence of the fascination with fitness. The new focus on the body was particularly evident in books and videos, as celebrities young and old told the secrets of their physical fitness regimens: Raquel Welch, John Travolta, Linda Evans, Victoria Principal, Jayne Kennedy, Marie Osmond, and, most famously, Jane Fonda, were just a few of the stars who produced exercise guides, videos, or both.[88] Lifestyle fitness magazines became more popular than ever. Entrepreneur Joe Weider's stable of publications—Muscle and Fitness, Shape, Flex, and Sports Fitness—were selling almost 2 million copies a month combined.[89] By 1984, sales for the fitness industry amounted to $900 million—an increase of 33 percent over the previous year—and that figure didn't include books, videos, or an estimated $500 million in sales of fitness apparel.[90]

Intense workouts and visible musculature were part of a new fitness ethos grounded in toughness. This was radically different from the easy-going jogging culture of a decade earlier. Fitness culture in the 1980s seemed to take its cues from political culture. The Reagan presidency embraced militarism, staunch anticommunism, and free enterprise, and it ushered in a new kind of fitness that made no apologies for its mentality of dominance.[91] The president's promotion of his exercise regimen in *Parade* magazine was emblematic of the cultural turn that exercise had taken. Historian Kenneth Dutton has noted the political overtones that characterized the muscular bodies of the 1980s and the not-so-muscular ones of the previous decade. The bony, long-haired, emaciated figures that typified protesters' physiques, epitomized by musicians David Bowie and Mick Jagger, had been abandoned for a new muscular ideal that denoted "patriotic heroism, physical power and even militarism."[92] The long, lean bodies of joggers had more in common with Bowie and Jagger than with weight lifters. It was this association that made Jimmy Carter's failed ten-kilometer run so significant; when a critic charged that jogging was not "presidential," he hinted at a perception of jogging as nonconformist, countercultural, and weak.[93]

Reagan recognized that muscles *were* presidential. His understanding of symbols that conveyed a sense of might produced a discourse of hard and soft bodies that bore striking similarities to fitness discussions during the early Cold War. Film historian Susan Jeffords has made a compelling argument that Reagan privileged a normative body that "enveloped strength, labor, determination, loyalty and courage."[94] Illustrating how this ethos was depicted on film, she has shown that the sculpted, muscular body was used as a symbol of dominance in the character of John Rambo, hero of a three-film series that paralleled Reagan's two terms.[95] The extent to which the president was identified with the Rambo character, played by actor Sylvester Stallone, was made clear by Reagan's nickname: Ronbo.[96] Reagan brought to office a rhetoric of uplift that he believed would address the national feelings of shame and guilt he described as the "Vietnam Syndrome." Rambo, a Vietnam veteran, must return to that country in the first film to rescue prisoners of war, allowing a 1980s reworking of the war and a second chance at victory onscreen and in U.S. popular culture.

Even though she mentions fitness trends only in passing, Jeffords's argument, and the films she discusses, would not have been possible were it not for the aesthetic style popularized by gay men and bodybuilders. The victory culture that Reagan espoused infused fitness culture with a new sense of power and a reinvigoration of the virtues associated with hard bodies: self-mastery, upward mobility, and discipline. No longer was it enough to go for a three-mile jog or play a friendly game of tennis a few times a week. Exercise in the 1980s was labor-intensive. The turn toward strenuosity began in the late 1970s as "jogging" gradually transitioned to "running." In 1982, the *Runner* looked back on the evolution of jogging over the previous decade. In a chart that tracked training and terminology shifts, Hal Higdon showed how mileage, goals, and motivation had changed over time. In 1972, health was the motivating factor, with joggers logging from five to fifteen miles weekly; in 1977, finishing a marathon had become the new goal, and weekly mileage had increased to thirty to fifty miles. By 1982, runners were completing upwards of fifty miles a week, and fitness had become a competitive pursuit.[97] The Ironman Triathlon, for example, got its start in 1978, and within a few years it had grown to several hundred participants, warranting live television coverage.[98] Exercise in the 1980s meant making measurable gains (or losses), pushing the limits of one's physical endurance, and setting personal bests. The mantra "No pain, no gain" became ubiquitous. Even aerobics, which had initially been infused with a joyous sense of movement, turned hard core, with marathon sessions, ballistic movements, and music loud enough to cause hearing damage. Jane Fonda's infamous mantra "Feel the burn" was evidence of the shift from physical liberation and heart health to hard labor and accomplishment.[99]

This ethos was on display in the workplace, where visible musculature was worn like a suit of armor. Bodies became tools to intimidate competitors and foster self-confidence. As one Houston banker attested, "If I'm working with or competing with someone who's really out of shape, I feel like I can do a better job than he."[100] Not caring about one's health—which was increasingly conflated with appearance—had become a form of deviance. In her study of the lives of what she termed the "singular generation"—twenty-something adults of the 1980s—author Wanda Urbanska related a conversation between two women overheard at a California gym. As one described the positive qualities of the man she had recently begun to date, she complained, "The only thing about him is he will not work out. He flat out refuses." Her workout partner replied, "So you're going to have to let him go." "Do I have a choice?" she sighed.[101]

CREATING COMMUNITY AT THE GYM

Perhaps the most enduring legacy of the 1980s in terms of fitness trends is not the type, duration, or intensity of a particular kind of workout but the fact that so many people came together regularly in a leisure setting. During the late 1970s and 1980s, the gym became a significant site of social exchange in American life. In 1989, sociologist Ray Oldenburg published *The Great Good Place*, lamenting the demise of "third places." With home and work representing the first and second places, Oldenburg defined a third place as one that was close to home, required regular attendance, and provided a playful atmosphere as well as a familiar "home away from home" feeling. According to Oldenburg, places such as taverns, coffeehouses, or even the main street in a small town allowed for an informal public life and played a beneficial role in personal, political, and civil life by providing space for social interaction and a sense of belonging. Without them, he argued, citizens risked social isolation, a lack of community, and a stilted political and intellectual life.[102]

Written at the height of the fitness movement, *The Great Good Place* surprisingly never considered the gym as a third place.[103] By 1988, there were more than 15,000 commercial health clubs in the United States.[104] As a social center, the gym became a new kind of urban or suburban country club. Friendships and social connections were enabled because members believed that their fellow exercisers shared common interests and were likely to have a similar economic status and lifestyle. The near-daily demands of an exercise routine meant that relationships could build gradually over time. Members with the same exercise class preferences or workout schedules saw one another repeatedly, creating a kind of critical social mass on which to build friendships. Even if members' relationships never went beyond the gym's reception desk, the sense of permanence, regularity, and routine provided by the gym created a sense of belonging and community, which, Oldenburg argues, is crucial to the creation of a third place. One California gym owner unknowingly employed Oldenburg's own terminology when he told a journalist in 1981, "Now, instead of going to the neighborhood tavern or someplace unhealthy, you go to a health club." Another lifelong gym member noted the change that had occurred in gyms, joking, "It's still two or two and a half hours from entering to leaving. However, actual exercise time is only 30 to 45 minutes, while an hour and a half is spent in the lounge making friends, meeting members of the opposite sex and seeking job leads."[105]

Club owners quickly recognized that the social aspects of membership were important to growing their businesses. Gyms in the 1980s often featured a full slate of social activities that extended beyond the purview of exercise. Some clubs routinely organized outside activities such as group vacations, day trips, and social hours.[106] Inside the gym space, facilities often included full-service restaurants, juice bars, and cocktail bars, all of which promoted member socialization.

Clubs in the 1980s grew increasingly larger in urban and suburban areas, in terms of both membership and square footage. Membership rosters numbering in the thousands were not uncommon, and amenities expanded to include beauty salons, nurseries, and spa services. Larger gyms in urban areas were just as well known as fine restaurants; newspapers and local-market magazines regularly ran features on the city's best places to work out.[107] Chicago's East Bank Club, the New York Health and Racquet Club, New York's Vertical Club, and the San Francisco Bay Club were among the elite clubs mentioned in national media outlets. Although smaller suburban health clubs may have offered fewer amenities, they provided the same kind of meeting ground to establish business contacts, make friends, and find lovers. A manager at a Santa Monica gym estimated that 80 percent of his patrons came to socialize and work out in equal measure, with only 20 percent looking for a serious workout alone.[108]

The same atmosphere that was conducive to building friendships also encouraged romantic relationships. Health clubs, the media breathlessly reported, had quickly replaced singles bars as the meeting place of the 1980s. Exercisers favorably compared gyms to bars, noting that the hard work of exercise made it easier to approach others. As a New York club employee put it, "It lowers barriers when everyone's groaning together."[109] A Washington, D.C., gym manager pointed out that opportunities to socialize were built into the club experience: "It's a lot easier to meet someone in this setting and say to them, 'Hey, let's go play racquetball tomorrow' than to lean over on a bar stool and say 'Let's go to my house.'"[110] Club members viewed their fellow exercisers as similar to themselves, using the club membership process as a type of screening. The physical space of the gym was particularly important for women, who felt safer in a controlled, brightly lit atmosphere.[111]

In the gay community, health clubs were a linchpin of social life. The gym was important both for the bodies it molded and for the social and romantic opportunities it presented. As one man summed up the era, "In the early 80s the gym was well on its way to replacing the bar as the central institution of gay life for a large number of guys in New York City. For many of us the gym had become a kind of community center, the hub of overlapping circles of friendship, sex and romance."[112]

In the late 1970s, sociologist Martin Levine documented the social world of gay clone culture in urban centers. He reported that men's social networks were based almost exclusively on cliques or same-sex friendship circles that traveled an established though variable loop of bars, restaurants, discos, and gyms.[113] As an integral element of the social network, gyms were a frequent meeting spot for gay men who traveled the "circuit." The gym was as much a site for social encounters as were local bars and discos. In 1978, John Blair, owner of the Bodycenter, the first gym in Manhattan to target an exclusively gay clientele, solicited members by going to Studio 54 and handing out gym passes "to every cute boy around."[114] Similarly, Chelsea Gym, another gay-owned facility, first advertised for members in the newsletter of the Saint, a well-known nightclub.[115] Much like bars and clubs of the period, the popularity of a particular gym could wax and wane, depending on its novelty and membership. One circuit traveler chronicled the ups and downs of the New York gym scene in the early 1980s, noting that "when the Bodycenter first opened it was 'hot.' Everyone left the New York Health Club on Thirteenth Street for the Bodycenter. The crowd has now moved to the Chelsea Gym and the Bodycenter is tired."[116] Though the specific location was subject to change, maintaining a gym membership was a given for men who frequented the circuit.

Seventies clone culture valued the gym-built body primarily for aesthetic reasons. The arrival of AIDS in the following decade, however, led to a radical shift in the significance of the gym routine. One of the distinguishing characteristics of AIDS was a gaunt, wasted appearance. Strength training countered this by creating and maintaining muscle mass, which not only disguised the disease's visible effects but also provided a measure of defense against its wasting process. One AIDS sufferer attributed his continuing good health to his gym habit: "One of the reasons that I'm still healthy is my vanity," he explained. "That's why I work out—not for all the 'good' reasons. The gym taught me what feeling healthy felt like, and that was useful when I got sick. . . . And for people with AIDS, muscle mass is money in the bank."[117]

For both the healthy and the stricken, the act of working out and the muscular body it created were ways to resist this terrible disease. Adhering to a workout routine allowed men to maintain a measure of control over their bodies and to affirm the physical liberation achieved by gay men in the years after Stonewall. As author Michaelangelo Signorile explained, "Being healthy and disease-free also began to mean having muscles and a strong, sturdy body. . . . We were out to prove we were supermen despite AIDS."[118]

AIDS brought a number of changes to the social lives of gay men in urban areas. Bathhouses quickly closed for fear of contagion, but other institutions also experienced a downturn as the community hunkered down. Men's social lives focused increasingly on the home, and as a result, attendance at gay bars and discos declined.[119] This trend did not affect health clubs, however. "Rather than going to the bar for happy hour, people are meeting their friends at the health club," a Brooklyn business owner observed.[120] In the absence of other venues, gyms became even more important as sites of community. At New York's Chelsea Gym, one of the city's best-known men-only health clubs, members reported that it was not unusual to see men recently released from the hospital, some with lesions from Kaposi's sarcoma, others with catheters attached to their chests, still exercising just days before death.[121] The friendships formed at the gym helped cement the social networks that carried men through this difficult period. Countering the belief that relationships formed at the gym were somehow less solid than those made elsewhere, one man explained, "The notion that these circles of gym buddies and disco friends would be scattered by the first winds of winter proved utterly untrue. These were the men who appeared in hospital rooms to rally round sick friends, creating ad hoc care groups that were remarkably effective."[122] After the loss of his partner, his gym friends provided support. "I was literally inundated by men expressing condolences and inquiring about how I was doing when I returned to the gym. Some were not even people I was friends with, but rather had only known to say hello to on the floor of the gym. No one seemed to mind when I broke down in tears telling a story about a particular part of his dying."[123]

While critics such as Oldenburg have charged that American society has become increasingly fragmented and less community oriented, gyms, in their capacity as membership organizations, appear to counter this trend.[124] On arriving in a new town or even a new neighborhood, finding a health club is near the top of the to-do list for many people.

The Business of Fitness

While gyms became sites of community during the 1980s, the fitness industry has not always been so welcoming or even ethical in its business dealings. The nature of the club model of business, as well as the redefinition of gym space as one grounded in glamour and affluence, meant that gyms promoted, intentionally and unintentionally, a sense of exclusivity. For much of the industry's history, this translated to membership discrimination. Deceptive or fraudulent business practices were also a problem, especially in the early years as business models evolved. New chains often promised more than they could provide, and customers who bought "lifetime memberships" sometimes arrived for a workout only to find locked doors when a club suddenly went bankrupt.

While the 1950s and 1960s saw the gentrification of the gym space, gyms' business practices were a work in progress at best. Chains of the era often expanded rapidly but became insolvent just as fast. Overly aggressive sales techniques on the part of some clubs also lent an air of ill repute to the industry, despite the gym's modernized interior. By 1962, Vic Tanny's Gym and Health Club had eighty-eight properties that grossed $35 million annually, but sales were often generated by high-pressure tactics and exaggerated claims of physical improvement. Tanny once famously authored a sales script for staff members that concluded, "If you fail to get an appointment (for a club tour and in-person sales pitch), then take a gun out of the desk and shoot yourself."[125] Anecdotes abounded about membership consultants who resorted to drastic measures to get a potential member to sign a contract; one woman charged that she had been held hostage in a manager's office until she agreed.[126] In a single three-month period, Tanny sales staff reportedly obtained membership contracts totaling $9 million.[127] Even so, the rate at which membership dues were paid could not keep pace with the high overhead costs. Problems attributed to "too rapid expansion, inadequate capital and management errors" led to the chain's seizure by creditors in 1962. Club closings stranded members who had paid large sums for "lifetime privileges." In addition, owing to the nature of the contract, many creditors continued to request payment from members even after the gyms closed.[128] Many of the Tanny locations were bought out by new, smaller entities and reopened. The company's demise was widely reported by the national media; surprisingly, in spite of Tanny's tarnished image, some of the new owners chose to maintain the Tanny name.[129]

Reducing salon chains were no different. Slenderella's rapid expansion launched it onto a similar path of financial ruin. The company failed to pay over $1 million in federal taxes, leading IRS agents to raid its salons in 1959, seizing cash, closing facilities, and leaving women who had prepaid for session packages with no financial recourse.[130] A 1962 episode of the television show The Green Hornet, set in the fictitious Vale of Eden health club, depicted a Slenderella-like salon where male and female patrons listened to "special" music during treatments, which brainwashed them into unknowingly committing crimes.[131] The show hinted at the unseemly side of the fitness business and illustrated that consumers, though enticed by its claims, remained somewhat distrustful of its promises to reshape their bodies.

Overzealous claims of effectiveness and unscrupulous business practices, such as those engaged in by Slenderella and Tanny, tarnished the fitness industry and left it with a less than wholesome reputation. This reputation continued to dog the industry through the 1970s and 1980s. The club model allowed a proprietor to set up shop with minimal expenditures because the equipment and space were typically leased; once in operation, the business became dependent on membership sales for cash flow. "Health clubs have become a wonderful way for people with very little capital to defraud the small consumer," a California prosecutor charged.[132] Consumer protection agencies were often called in when members who had prepurchased services lost substantial sums of money. By the mid-1970s, federal and state authorities began to investigate what regulators called the health spa industry. The federal pursuit of industry-wide regulation lasted a decade but was eventually abandoned in 1985 during the Reagan administration. By 1987, however, twenty-seven states had enacted consumer protection laws requiring "cooling-off periods" or the ability to break a contract shortly after signing, as well as redress mechanisms for closed clubs, such as requiring bonds from business owners.[133]

The sense of exclusivity that health clubs cultivated through chrome weights, well-appointed locker rooms, and thick carpeting often extended to their membership rolls. From the industry's early years and continuing through the 1980s, clubs, including the YMCA, discriminated against nonwhite potential members. Taking their cues from country clubs, both commercial and nonprofit clubs worked to ensure that their membership was composed of "desirable clients." YMCA BMCs, for example, admittedly engaged in racial and religious profiling to ensure a "proper balance" among members. A survey of membership practices in the 1940s revealed that about 40 percent of clubs required some sort of screening process before admitting a new member. Race, religion, age, and occupation were factors used to determine whether to accept a new member; nineteen clubs had a whites-only policy, and fifteen other clubs "maintained a limit of not over 10 per cent Hebrew."[134] Segregationist policies continued through the 1950s and 1960s at Y locations and in commercial health clubs. In 1959, for example, an African American member of the Philadelphia YMCA's board of directors resigned in protest of the decision to "hold" his application for membership in the health club for later consideration; Marshall L. Sheppard described the Y's decision as segregationist. Y leadership denied the allegation, noting that the health club already had one African American member.[135] Two years later, Dr. Eugene Reed visited a Vic Tanny gym on Long Island. Reed was told that the club had a long waiting list for membership, but a white friend who applied to join shortly after Reed was quickly enrolled. Reed, president of the New York NAACP, brought suit against the chain, and the case was settled shortly before it went before the state supreme court.[136] In 1967, a traveling jazz pianist who was a member of the Y near his home in California was refused entrance to the Atlanta Y while visiting that city on tour. Les McCann was "shocked and angered to find that a so-called Christian association" would deny him access. Although the Atlanta Y itself was integrated, the health club was not; Atlanta leadership inexplicably cited the facility's near-full capacity as the reason for maintaining a segregated membership.[137] These reports signal an ongoing pattern of discrimination and likely represent only a fraction of the actual number of discriminatory episodes.

Racial discrimination continued through the 1980s. In 1989, the Justice Department filed a civil suit against U.S. Health (a subsidiary of Bally Manufacturing), which operated health clubs in Washington, Baltimore, Philadelphia, Boston, and Atlanta. It charged that employees were directed to discourage black customers from joining and quoted them higher rates and poorer credit terms than those offered to white customers. Additional suits were brought by groups of club members and employees who alleged that visits by prospective black members were coded in sales log books as "DNWAM," or "do not want as member." Employees who did not follow the company's membership practices were fired or harassed. In the Washington, D.C., area, sales consultants steered prospective black members to three predominantly black clubs. African American employees also charged that they were prohibited from working at the most affluent club locations. U.S. Health admitted guilt in 1991, and as part of a settlement agreement, it paid damages and offered free memberships to blacks who had paid inflated club rates or had been turned away. In addition, future club advertising was required to include images of blacks and a statement of its nondiscrimination policy. As a result of another suit, a fund was created to compensate African Americans who had sought employment with the chain but had been rejected because of their race.[138] These suits, along with the cultural profile of the typical exerciser as a white professional, explain the relative absence of African Americans from fitness trends of the 1980s, which led Sports Illustrated to observe in 1984, "You can scan hundreds of product catalogs, mail-order brochures, fitness magazines, books and videos and see nothing but attractive lily-white faces."[139]

THE LIMITS OF THE "BOOM"

Only a few years into the decade of vigorous exercise, fitness buffs were in pain. Injuries had become common; repetitive stress on feet and knees in high-impact aerobics classes was particularly damaging. One study found that more than 75 percent of instructors and 43 percent of participants had exercise-induced injuries.[140] Unqualified group fitness instructors and trainers also led to "health club victims."[141] The fitness industry had grown quickly, and it had few mechanisms in place to ensure quality control. Fewer than one in twenty instructors had a degree in exercise physiology or certification from the American College of Sports Medicine, the International Dance-Exercise Association, or the Aerobics and Fitness Association of America, which were among the first organizations to establish accreditation criteria for fitness professionals.[142]

The recognition that, when it came to exercise, one size did not fit all led to the development and introduction of new kinds of fitness classes and devices. Physicians were urging less intense workouts, and instructors responded with the creation of low-impact aerobics and classes incorporating elements from other types of exercise, such as martial arts and yoga.[143] The 1989 development of Reebok's step bench, a raised platform that replicated the act of climbing stairs and thus increased one's heart rate, was a result of the need for a safe but high-intensity workout.[144] New scientific research showed that health gains could also be derived from lower-intensity exercise, supporting this trend.[145] Moreover, the belief that regular, intense workouts could dramatically transform one's body seemed to fade as people realized that genetics simply couldn't be denied. While physical improvement was possible, total transformation was not. "The reality is we aren't all body beautifuls. Everybody can't be a Jane Fonda or an Arnold Schwarzenegger," one YMCA executive admitted.[146]

For most Americans, the 1980s brought a new awareness of the need for physical activity and the normalization of exercise as a form of leisure. The frenetic impulse to exercise gave way to the realization that the pursuit of fitness was best viewed as a lifetime habit. Near the end of the decade, there were signs that the fitness movement was waning. According to a study by the National Center for Health Statistics, overall participation in exercise and strenuous activity declined by 10 percent between 1985 and 1990, and exercise participants became slightly less active than in the recent past.[147] Although some evidence suggested that the decline in participation was attributable to a lack of free time among the most vigorous exercisers—baby boomers—additional studies showed that participation was declining across all age groups.[148] In spite of the considerable buzz about exercise, health clubs, and muscles, the U.S. Public Health Service still estimated that 80 to 90 percent of all Americans were not engaging in sufficient physical activity.[149] This suggests that the idea of fitness was more popular than the actual practice of exercise. It also indicates that a large swath of the population had been excluded from the fitness movement for reasons of cost, bias, time, or disinterest. Though some Americans had wholeheartedly embraced exercise, most had not. Even for the most enthusiastic exercisers, it was difficult to sustain the momentum of the 1980s.

In 1986, journalist Blair Sabol chronicled the ups and downs in fitness trends over the previous fifteen years. Expressing a sense of fatigue as the intense decade wound down, she observed that the strenuosity of the 1980s had been "a craze. And it was the craziness that became injurious to the entire health movement." Citing her own injuries and those of other athletes, she argued for moderation and unwittingly predicted the advent of yoga in the 1990s. "Basically, we all need a giant rest. We've pounded and pumped, humped, and dumped our physiques into a vacuum and now we need to get back to some sense of basics—to forms of moderate movement. . . . We need to experience that integration between physical coordination and mental awareness."[150] Exercise was about to come full circle in its embrace of more sedate forms of physical activity. Just thirty years earlier, it had seemed unlikely that vigorous physical activity would become the preferred hobby of middle-class men and women. Physical fitness had been a vague concept with little cultural capital and nearly no scientific backing. By the end of the 1980s, the aching bodies of baby boomers were evidence of exercise's ascendance, but also of its limited reach.

THE FUTURE OF FITNESS

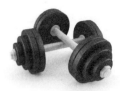

In 1968, antiexercise physician Peter Steincrohn predicted that when scholars set about writing the history of the twentieth century, exercise promotion would be one of its defining features—if not *the* defining element of the previous 100 years. In typical fashion, he lambasted the "pathetic beliefs of Americans in the need for special exercises and the need for special diets. These two oddities will overshadow miniskirts, guitars, scraggly beards—and perhaps the Bomb itself," he grimly surmised.[1] Steincrohn realized that a nation's beliefs about its collective well-being reveal profound truths about its culture and demonstrate that exercise is only rarely a simple act of recreation. The practice and discussion of fitness provide insight into how people negotiate their environment and their thoughts on health and appearance, work and leisure, and the factors that constitute a good life and even a good death.

As the research in this book has shown, the term *fitness* and the ways to achieve it are constantly being reexamined in light of developments in scientific research, trends in popular culture, and health promotion policies. The evolution of fitness is a process fraught with contradiction and contest. In the last two decades, new forms of physical activity have joined weight lifting, aerobics, and jogging to expand the realm of what most people understand as exercise. The recent rediscovery of yoga and Pilates has added to the growing list of qualities a fit person must possess.[2] A new emphasis on balance, flexibility, core strength, and stress reduction is evidenced by the growing attendance at yoga and Pilates classes in health clubs around the nation, not to mention at stand-alone studios. Perhaps this new attention to the "mind-body" connection—involving a type of mental fitness after all—would make PCYF director Shane MacCarthy smile.

These new fitness trends have influenced bodies as well. The muscular physiques of the 1980s and 1990s have ceded ground to leaner, more elongated, dance-inspired figures, proving that exercise has again made the body itself a fashion accessory. Unfortunately, these recent fitness developments continue to perpetuate the notion that exercise is an activity of the well-to-do. Classes at yoga studios tend to be even more expensive than gym memberships, and designer yoga apparel does nothing to dismantle this notion, in spite of the practice's humble core beliefs.[3] Yoga is well on its way to replacing (or at least joining) other forms of exercise as evidence of self-possession and interior mettle, much as jogging and company gym workouts did for male executives in the late 1960s. London's *Sunday Telegraph* recently observed, "In New York, the yoga capital of the Western world, the studio is fast replacing the private members' club, or golf club, as the place to be seen or steal 'face time' with people who you want to impress or give you a job," illustrating that even an activity developed to rid the self of ego can be reformulated as a conscious demonstration of self-presentation.[4] Yoga posing competitions—which some would call the antithesis of the practice—have even sprung up as yogis attempt to outdo one another.[5] In many ways, the appropriation of yoga in American culture resembles the trajectories of other forms of fitness. Marketers have exploited yoga's messages for profit, and consumers have adapted it for a multitude of purposes, some of which—such as Christian yoga—were never imagined by its Hindu creators.[6]

The formalization of exercise as a practice—a process that has taken place mainly through the lens of consumer culture—has made us much more serious about our exercise routines and, I would argue, has removed at least some of the pleasure from physical activity. As this book sketches out, the work ethic was largely absent from the practice of exercise at midcentury, but in the course of making exercise a legitimate use of leisure time, we have very consciously inserted it. Fitness in twenty-first-century America is highly structured and workmanlike. The relatively new focus on intensity and measurable improvement seems to suggest that corporeal pleasure alone can't justify one's participation in exercise. The idea that fitness can be achieved by sitting in a sauna, resting in a YMCA "nap room," or using an electrical device to whittle one's waist might seem laughable to us now, but these earlier conceptions of fitness are indicative of our present need to make leisure time as productive as work time, and perhaps they demonstrate the triumph of the market economy as well.[7] The development of fitness culture has transpired in near lockstep with the expansion of the white-collar workplace. Exercise was, and remains, a mode of ensuring one's readiness for work. The 1950s image of the harried, coronary-prone businessman who relied on pills and cocktails to get through the day has been replaced by the self-possessed, ultra-fit man or woman who can not only handle office stress with ease but also make time for triathlon training. The continued use of fitness to display our worthiness in the workplace illustrates how little value we attribute to leisure and relaxation, although the arrival of yoga on the fitness scene offers some hopeful signs.

Fitness culture relies on the premise that the solution to the nation's physical inactivity can be found in the individual, even though it's apparent that sedentary lifestyles are a societal problem. In the nineteenth century, participation in physical culture was legitimated by the fact that it served the common good. One reason that Shane MacCarthy's total fitness mission failed was because it appealed to obligation in a new era of individuality.[8] Calls to duty could no longer be heard over the din of popular culture's enjoinders to have fun and enjoy oneself. For a brief period in the early 1960s, fitness was marketed primarily as fun, but by 1968, this idea was fading as jogging, grounded in exercise physiology, redefined leisure as working at health. Today, we perceive health as a personal accomplishment and the natural result of a morally correct life, and we make little room for luck, genetics, or the environment in assessing our own bodies and others'.

Inherent in the use of fitness as a marker of personal competency is the way that fit bodies function as a marker of difference or even superiority.

Just as slimness became more desirable as Americans' weight began to increase nationwide, the manufactured gym body became coveted as more people occupied sedentary positions at work. Historically, Americans of color and lower socioeconomic classes have been excluded from fitness culture. And fitness entrepreneurs' attempts to legitimate exercise participation by marketing it as an exclusive, sought-after activity have constructed exercise as a luxury rather than as basic health maintenance. The health club model—based on the nineteenth-century athletic club, with its membership restrictions—has also contributed to this notion. It's evident that if we truly want all Americans to get moving, the belief that exercise is the province of a certain demographic group needs to be dismantled.

In spite of our modern fascination with fitness, a number of benchmarks indicate that exercise—at least as we now practice it—is not enough to make us healthy as a population. Less than half of all Americans meet recommended guidelines for cardiovascular physical activity, and only about 20 percent engage in both cardiovascular and muscle strengthening physical activity in recommended measures.[9] Busy schedules prohibit many people from devoting an hour a day to their bodies multiple times a week. And the costs associated with a fitness routine can be a barrier. These problems are compounded by the relatively narrow definition of exercise that has taken shape in American culture. To most people, exercising requires substantial overhead: special clothing, a lengthy block of time, and a designated workout space. In the absence of any of these factors, people often choose to do nothing—when, in fact, a twenty-minute walk around the block would have been a healthy choice. This somewhat grim assessment of fitness culture, however, shouldn't obscure the many benefits that enthusiastic exercisers derive from their fitness routines. For a relatively small group of people, exercise has been and continues to be a powerful force in shaping lifestyles and positively influencing health.

The lifestyle changes that mid-twentieth-century Americans first noticed have continued unabated. Physical activity is declining in all aspects of American life—at work, at home, and in our commutes. The one exception is leisure time, likely due to persistent exercise promotion efforts.[10] Even as our romance with fitness culture expands into new realms of activity, it's clear that working out a few times a week is not sufficient to counteract the sedentary nature of our technology-driven, automobile-dependent existence. We need to find new ways to put moderate amounts of energy expenditure back into our daily lives, and this will require significant changes in planning and land use, modes of travel, and architecture, along with a dose of unconventionality. In public health and medicine, research into the role of physical activity outside the framework of exercise is growing. The phrase *nonexercise activity thermogenesis*, coined by physician James Levine, is based on his belief that the cumulative health effects of a "chair-based" or "desk-bound" lifestyle (as Americans of the 1950s would have put it) cannot be undone by a few workouts a week. Increasingly, scientists are finding that the sedentary nature of life in modern America can be just as unhealthy as the lack of vigorous physical activity. New attention to the dangers of prolonged sitting, for example, has led to the invention of the treadmill desk, an out-of-the-box method of putting physicality back into sedentary forms of labor.[11]

The need for better solutions to the problem of the body in modern culture is becoming more critical as the problem expands worldwide. The environmental and lifestyle changes that midcentury Americans observed are now unfolding in many developing nations. In China, Brazil, and India, where fast-growing economies are now raising the comfort levels of millions of citizens, the increasingly sedentary nature of life "represents a major threat to global health." Shu Wen Ng and Barry Popkin's recent study of global trends in physical activity in leisure, work, transportation, and the domestic sphere suggests that twentieth-century critics of American affluence were on the mark in their warnings about the hazards of modern conveniences. Based on current activity patterns, Ng and Popkin predict that threats to cardiometabolic health will become more severe over time.[12] Given the grand scale of this growing problem, it's evident that the incompatibility of our bodies and our lifestyles will be rectified only through population-wide solutions, not personal health revolutions.

NOTES

Introduction: Fitness in American Culture

1. Donald Dukelow, "A Doctor Looks at Exercise and Fitness,"*Journal of Health, Physical Education, Recreation* 6 (1957): 24–26.

2. American College of Sports Medicine, "Recommended Quantity and Quality of Exercise for Developing and Maintaining Fitness in Healthy Adults," *Medicine in Sport Science* 10 (1978): vii–x.

3. Steven Findlay, "Smart Ways to Shape Up," *U.S. News & World Report*, July 18, 1988, 46–49.

4. Alton Blakeslee and Jeremiah Stamler, *Your Heart Has Nine Lives* (New York: Pocket Books, 1963), 7.

5. "Obesity Is Now No. 1 U.S. Nutritional Problem," *Science News Letter*, December 27, 1952, 408; Bess Furman, "Obesity Is Termed No. 1 Nutritional Ill," *New York Times*, December 9, 1952, 45.

6. Hans Kraus and Ruth P. Hirschland, "Muscular Fitness and Health," *Journal of Health, Physical Education, Recreation* 24, 10 (1953): 17–19.

7. See, for example, Elaine Tyler May, *Homeward Bound: American Families in the Cold War Era* (New York: Basic Books, 1988); Andrew Wiese, *Places of Their Own: African American Suburbanization in the Twentieth Century* (Chicago: University of Chicago Press, 2004); Lizabeth Cohen, *A Consumer's Republic: The Politics of Mass Consumption in Postwar America* (New York: Knopf, 2003); Thomas Hine, *Populuxe* (New York: Knopf, 1986); Kenneth T. Jackson, *Crabgrass Frontier: The Suburbanization of the United States* (Oxford: Oxford University Press, 1985).

8. "The Impact of the Built Environment on Health: An Emerging Field," *American Journal of Health Promotion* 93, 9 (September 2003): 1382–1384; Alyson Geller, "Smart Growth: A Prescription for Livable Cities," *American Journal of Health Promotion* 93, 9 (September 2003): 1410–1414.

9. Reid Ewing, "The Relationship between Urban Sprawl, Physical Activity, Obesity and Morbidity," *American Journal of Health Promotion* 18, 1 (September–October 2003): 47–57. See also Rob Stein, "Suburbia USA: Fat of the Land?"*Washington Post*, August 29, 2003, A3.

10. The lack of long-term data makes it difficult to track physical activity patterns; however, researchers have been able to conclude that in most aspects of life, physical activity has been in decline since the 1950s. Ross C. Brownson, Tegan K. Boehmer, and Douglas A. Luke, "Declining Rates of Physical Activity in the United States: What Are the Contributors?" *Annual Review of Public Health* 26 (2005): 421–443.

11. Nancy Struna, *People of Prowess: Sport, Leisure, and Labor in Early Anglo-America* (Urbana: University of Illinois, 1996); Benjamin G. Rader, *American Sports: From the Age of Folk Games to the Age of Televised Sports* (Upper Saddle River, N.J.: Prentice Hall, 1983); Stephen Nissenbaum, *Sex, Diet and Debility in Jacksonian America: Sylvester Graham and Health Reform* (Westport, Conn.: Greenwood, 1980); Martha Verbrugge, *Able Bodied Womanhood: Personal Health and Social Change in 19th Century Boston* (New York: Oxford University Press, 1988); Clifford W. Putney, *Muscular Christianity: Manhood and Sports in Protestant America, 1880–1920* (Cambridge, Mass.: Harvard University Press, 2001); Donald J. Mrozek, *Sport and American Mentality, 1880–1910* (Knoxville: University of Tennessee Press, 1983); James Whorton, *Crusaders for Fitness: The History of American Health Reformers* (Princeton, N.J.: Princeton University Press, 1982); Robert Ernst, *Weakness Is a Crime: The Life of Bernarr MacFadden* (Syracuse, N.Y.: Syracuse University Press, 1991); John Kasson, *Houdini, Tarzan and the Perfect Man: The White Male Body and the Challenge of Modernity in America* (New York: Hill & Wang, 2001); William R. Hunt, *Body Love: The Amazing Career of Bernarr MacFadden* (Bowling Green, Ohio: Bowling Green University Popular Press, 1989); Harvey Green, *Fit for America: Health, Fitness, Sport and American Society* (Baltimore: Johns Hopkins University Press, 1988); Gail Bederman, *Manliness and Civilization: A Cultural History of Race and Gender in the United States, 1880–1917* (Chicago: University of Chicago Press, 1995); David Kaufman, *Shul with a Pool: The Synagogue Center in America* (Hanover, N.H.: University Press of New England, 1999); Kristin Hoganson, *Fighting for American Manhood: How Gender Politics Provoked the Spanish American and Philippine American Wars* (New Haven, Conn.: Yale University Press, 1998); Linda J. Borish, "The Robust Woman and the Muscular Christian: Catherine Beecher, Thomas Higginson, and Their Vision of American Society, Health, and Physical Actitivites," *The International Journal of the History of Sport* 4 (September 1987): 139–154; *Fit: Episodes in the History of the Body*, directed by Laurie Block, Straight Ahead Pictures, 1991; Jan Todd, *Physical Culture and the Body Beautiful: Purposive Exercise in the Lives of American Women, 1800–1870* (Macon, GA: Mercer University Press).

12. Warren Susman, *Culture as History: The Transformation of American Society in the Twentieth Century* (New York: Pantheon, 1984).

13. Peter Bunzel, "Health Kick's High Priest," *Life*, September 29, 1958, 73; Dominique Padurano, "Making American Men: Charles Atlas and the Business of Bodies, 1892–1945" (Ph.D. diss., Rutgers University, 2007), 91–92, 158; "Helpmate for Herenow," *Newsweek*, July 25, 1960, 102.

14. Mark Adams, *Mr. America: How Muscular Millionaire Bernarr MacFadden Transformed the Nation through Sex, Salad, and the Ultimate Starvation Diet* (New York: HarperCollins, 2009); Padurano, "Making American Men"; Hunt, *Body Love*; Elizabeth Toon and Janet Golden, "'Live Clean, Think Clean, and Don't Go to Burlesque

Shows': Charles Atlas as Health Advisor," *Journal of the History of Medicine* 57 (January 2002): 39–60; Ernst, *Weakness Is a Crime*; Christina S. Jarvis, *The Male Body at War: American Masculinity during World War II* (De Kalb: Northern Illinois University Press, 2004); Roberta Park, *Measurement of Physical Fitness: A Historical Perspective* (Washington, D.C.: U.S. Department of Health and Human Services, Public Health Service, 1988).

15. Patricia A. Eisenman and C. Robert Barnett, "Physical Fitness in the 1950s and 1970s: Why Did One Fail and the Other Boom?" *Quest* 31, 1 (1979): 114–122; Randy Roberts and James S. Olson, "Perfect Bodies, Eternal Youth: The Obsession of Modern America," *Lamar Journal of the Humanities* 25, 1 (1989): 39–55; Benjamin G. Rader, "The Quest for Self-Sufficiency and the New Strenuosity: Reflections on the Strenuous Life of the 1970s and 1980s," *Journal of Sport History* 18, 2 (Summer 1991): 255–266; Ruth Clifford Engs, *Clean Living Movements: American Cycles of Health Reform* (Westport, Conn.: Praeger, 2000); Thomas Stephens, "Secular Trends in Adult Physical Activity: Exercise Boom or Bust?" *Research Quarterly for Exercise and Sport* 58, 2 (1987): 94–105.

16. Harvey Green notes that, at least in earlier years, works on physical culture were typically second or third books written by tenured scholars with the freedom to choose their topics—including those that might not be taken seriously by their peers. Harvey Green, introduction to *Fitness in American Culture: Images of Health, Sport and the Body, 1830–1940*, ed. Kathryn Grover (Rochester, N.Y.: Margaret Woodbury Strong Museum, 1989), 3–4.

17. Kenneth Cooper, *Aerobics* (New York: M. Evans, 1968).

18. Park, *Measurement of Physical Fitness*; Russell R. Pate, "The Evolving Definition of Physical Fitness," *Quest* 40 (1988): 174–179.

19. Robert Reinhold, "Has the Aerobics Movement Peaked? An Interview with Ken Cooper," *New York Times Magazine*, March 29, 1987, 14.

20. Muriel R. Gillick, "Health Promotion, Jogging, and the Pursuit of the Moral Life," *Journal of Health Politics, Policy and Law* 9, 3 (Fall 1984): 369–387. On the medicalization of American culture, see Philip G. White, Kevin Young, and James Gillett, "Bodywork as a Moral Imperative: Some Critical Notes on Health and Fitness," *Loisir et Société* 18, 1 (1995): 159–182; Robert Crawford, "Individual Responsibility and Health Politics in the 1970s," in *Health Care in America*, ed. Susan Reverby and David Rosner (Philadelphia: Temple University Press, 1979), 247–268; Robert Crawford, "You Are Dangerous to Your Health," *Social Policy* 8, 1 (January–February 1978): 11–20.

21. Jonathan M. Metzl, "Why 'Against Health'?" in *Against Health: How Health Became the New Morality*, ed. Jonathan M. Metzl and Anna Kirkland (New York: New York University, 2010), 2.

22. Ibid., 1–2.

23. Myra MacPherson, "Train (Pant, Pant) Don't Strain (Pant, Pant)," *New York Times*, February 13, 1968, 50.

24. *CBS Reports: The Fat American*, aired January 18, 1962.

25. National Center for Health Statistics, *Health, United States: With Special Feature on Socioeconomic Status and Health* (Hyattsville, Md.: National Center for Health Statistics, 2011), 272–276.

26. Eun-Ok Im et al., "'Physical Activity as a Luxury': African American Women's Attitudes toward Physical Activity," *Western Journal of Nursing Research* 34, 3 (2012): 317–339.

27. Researcher Brian Wansink has published widely on human behavior and food decisions. He argues that Americans cannot accurately gauge their food needs because of the proliferation of food advertising, encouraging persistent eating. For a compendium of his studies, see Brian L. Wansink, *Mindless Eating: Why We Eat More Than We Think* (New York: Bantam, 2006). According to nutritionist Marion Nestle, federal agricultural policies promote unhealthy eating habits. Federal nutritional guidelines are reluctant to advocate reduced consumption of any product for fear of decreasing industry profit margins. See Marion Nestle, *Food Politics: How the Food Industry Influences Nutrition and Health* (Berkeley: University of California Press, 2002).

CHAPTER 1. "FITNESS BEGINS IN THE HIGH CHAIR"

1. Hans Kraus and Ruth P. Hirschland, "Muscular Fitness and Health," *Journal of Health, Physical Education, Recreation* 24, 10 (1953): 17–19. Their findings were also published as "Muscular Fitness and Orthopedic Disability," *New York State Journal of Medicine* 54 (1954): 212–215; and "Minimum Muscular Fitness Tests in School Children," *Research Quarterly* 25 (1954): 178–188.

2. Kraus and Hirschland, "Muscular Fitness and Health," 18.

3. Harry Henderson, "Are We and Our Children Getting Too Soft?" *Cosmopolitan*, August 1954, 16–22; Elizabeth Pope, "How Fit Are Our Children?" *Ladies' Home Journal*, March 1954, 69, 90–93; "Are We Becoming Soft? Why the President Is Worried about Our Fitness," *Newsweek*, September 26, 1955, 35–36. See also "What's Wrong with American Youths," *U.S. News & World Report*, March 19, 1954, 35–36; "Why Are Americans' Muscles Getting Flabby?" *San Diego Union*, September 25, 1955, C2.

4. Even works that recognize the crisis sparked by the Kraus-Hirschland study fail to note the importance of the PCYF or see its work as distinct from the President's Council on Physical Fitness under Kennedy. See, for example, Robert L. Griswold, "The 'Flabby American,' the Body, and the Cold War," in *A Shared Experience: Men, Women and the History of Gender*, ed. Laura Mccall and Donald Yacovone

(New York: New York University Press, 1998), 323–348; Jeffrey Montez de Oca, "'As Our Muscles Get Softer, Our Missile Race Becomes Harder': Cultural Citizenship and the Muscle Gap," *Journal of Historical Sociology* 18, 3 (September 2005): 145–172; Donald J. Mrozek, "The Cult and Ritual of Toughness in Cold War America," in *Rituals and Ceremonies in Popular Culture*, ed. Ray B. Browne (Bowling Green, Ohio: Bowling Green University Popular Press, 1980), 178–191; Randy Roberts and James S. Olson, "Perfect Bodies, Eternal Youth: The Obsession of Modern America," *Lamar Journal of the Humanities* 25, 1 (1989): 39–55; Marc Richards, "The Cold War's 'Soft' Recruits," *Peace Review* 10, 3 (September 1998): 435–441; David W. Zang, *Sports Wars: Athletes in the Age of Aquarius* (Fayetteville: University of Arkansas Press, 2001), 74.

5. *Fitness of American Youth: A Report to the President of the United States on the President's Conference on Fitness of American Youth* (Washington, D.C.: U.S. Government Printing Office, 1956), 4.

6. "Are We Becoming Soft?" 35–36.

7. The term *push-button gadget* stems from the midcentury period, when electronic devices and appliances became markedly more complicated. Historian Susan Strasser notes that, by the 1960s, gadgets that had once been simply switched on and off were gradually being transformed into miracles of technology, with multiple buttons and more complicated features. Susan Strasser, *Never Done: A History of American Housework*, 2nd ed. (New York: Henry Holt, 2000), 279–280.

8. Barbara Melosh, *Engendering Culture: Manhood and Womanhood in New Deal Public Art and Theater* (Washington, D.C.: Smithsonian Institution Press, 1991).

9. Christina S. Jarvis, *The Male Body at War: American Masculinity during World War II* (De Kalb: Northern Illinois University Press, 2004).

10. Paul Starr, *The Social Transformation of American Medicine* (New York: Basic Books, 1982), 335–351; James H. Cassedy, *Medicine in America: A Short History* (Baltimore: Johns Hopkins University Press, 1991), 125–134; Joseph E. Illick, *American Childhoods* (Philadelphia: University of Pennsylvania Press, 2002), 113–114.

11. John B. Kelly, "Are We Becoming a Nation of Weaklings?" *Reader's Digest*, July 1956, 27.

12. David Masci, "Baby Boomers at Midlife," *CQ Researcher* 8, 28 (1998): 649–672.

13. James Gilbert, *A Cycle of Outrage: America's Reaction to the Juvenile Delinquent in the 1950s* (New York: Oxford University Press, 1986), 14.

14. Ralph W. England Jr., "A Theory of Middle Class Juvenile Delinquency," *Journal of Criminal Law, Criminology and Police Science* 50, 6 (1960): 535.

15. Gilbert, *A Cycle of Outrage*, 63.

16. Ibid.

17. *Rebel without a Cause*, directed by Nicholas Ray, Warner Bros. Pictures, 1955;

Blackboard Jungle, directed by Richard Brooks, MGM Pictures, 1955; *Teen-Age Crime Wave*, directed by Fred F. Sears, Columbia Pictures, 1955; *Crime in the Streets*, directed by Don Siegel, Allied Artists, 1956; *The Delinquents*, directed by Robert Altman, United Artists, 1957.

18. Gilbert, *A Cycle of Outrage*.

19 Eisenhower to Paul Hoy Helms, July 8, 1955, document 1501, Presidential Papers of Dwight David Eisenhower, http://www.eisenhowermemorial.org/menu.php?mid=36 (hereafter cited as Eisenhower Papers).

20. Jimmy Jemail, "Hotbox Special," *Sports Illustrated*, August 15, 1955, 32–33.

21. Richard Nixon to Betty R. Baldwin, July 25, 1955, Records of the President's Council on Physical Fitness, Department of Health, Education, and Welfare, Office of the Secretary, Correspondence and Reports, 1956–1968, National Archives, College Park, Md. (hereafter cited as PCPF Records).

22. Bob King to Richard Nixon, July 26, 1955, PCPF Records.

23. Eisenhower to Harley Cope, June 4, 1956, document 1887, Eisenhower Papers.

24. Although the focus on delinquency faded from the council's day-to-day workings, it continued to receive mention in annual reports as a reason to continue operations.

25. Henderson, "Are We and Our Children Getting Too Soft?" 16–22.

26. In 1954, Kraus spoke to the American Medical Association and the American Association for Health, Physical Education, and Recreation. See "US Children Fail in Muscle Tests," *New York Times*, April 24, 1954, 35; Susan E. B. Schwartz, *Into the Unknown: The Remarkable Life of Hans Kraus* (New York: iUniverse, 2005), 119. Prudden, a mountain-climbing partner of Kraus's, operated the Institute for Physical Fitness, a gymnastics and tumbling school for children in White Plains, N.Y. During the 1960s, she was one of the nation's leading fitness advocates. Later in life she developed "myotherapy," a pain-relieving technique employing pressure points. See Douglas Martin, "Bonnie Prudden, 97; Promoted Fitness for TV Generation," *New York Times*, December 19, 2011, B10.

27. *Fitness of American Youth: A Report to the President*, 17.

28. "Nixon to Head Study of Nation's Physique," *New York Times*, September 7, 1955, A1, 16.

29. "Talks on Fitness Open Tomorrow," *New York Times*, June 17, 1956, 45.

30. *Fitness of American Youth: A Report to the President*, 49–52.

31. *The American Catholic Who's Who* (Washington, D.C.: NC News Service, 1980), 457; "Pat on the Back: Shane MacCarthy," *Sports Illustrated*, October 1, 1956, 80.

32. Shane MacCarthy, "Enjoy Keeping Fit," *American Recreation Society Bulletin*, May 1957, 4–6.

33. To give one example of MacCarthy's busy travel schedule: during one ten-day period in fall 1959, MacCarthy either attended or addressed meetings at the Johnson Wax Company, the American Bicycle League of America, the Department of Defense Dependents Schools, the City of Buffalo, the American Podiatry Association, and the Catholic Chaplains' Correctional Association. *Fitness in Action* (PCYF newsletter), October 1959, PCPF Records.

34. "Special Report," undated (circa 1960), PCAC File, PCPF Records.

35. "A New Job for Nixon," *Pittsburgh Post*, September 10, 1955, clipping in PCPF Records.

36. President's Council on Youth Fitness, *Workshop Report No. 7: Sports for Fitness* (Washington, D.C.: U.S. Government Printing Office, 1960).

37. Gene Tunney to Shane MacCarthy, April 18, 1957, PCPF Records.

38. Fred Digby, "Ike Revives Fitness Plan," *Catholic Action of the South*, June 3, 1956, clipping in PCPF Records; Symon Gould to Vice President Richard Nixon, September 19, 1955, PCPF Records.

39. William Raab, University of Vermont, to Shane MacCarthy, March 8, 1959, PCPF Records.

40. President's Council on Youth Fitness, *Workshop Reports Nos. 2, 3 & 4: Communication Media, Magazine, Broadcasting* (Washington, D.C.: U.S. Government Printing Office, 1960), 5.

41. Dorothy Stull, "Conference at Annapolis: First Blow for Fitness," *Sports Illustrated*, July 2, 1956, 22–24.

42. U.S. Department of Health and Human Services, "Historical Background, Terminology, Evolution of Recommendations and Measurement," in *Physical Activity and Health: A Report of the Surgeon General* (Washington, D.C.: U.S. Government Printing Office, 1996), 15–16. Though scientists had long observed a correlation between exercise and longevity, it was not until the mid-1950s that a consensus based on scientific evidence was possible. See, for example, William J. Zukel et al., "A Short-Term Community Study of the Epidemiology of Coronary Heart Disease," *American Journal of Public Health* 49, 12 (1959): 1630–1639; William C. Pomeroy and Paul D. White, "Coronary Heart Disease in Former Football Players," *Journal of the American Medical Association* 167, 6 (1958): 711–714.

43. Dr. A. L. Chapman, chief of the Division of Special Health Services, Public Health Service, manuscript for "Speech at Health Program and Physical Education Workshop," Speeches, Programs, Reports File, PCPF Records.

44. Donald Dukelow, "A Doctor Looks at Exercise and Fitness," *Journal of Health, Physical Education, Recreation* 6 (1957): 24–26, 67.

45. William Walsh, M.D., to Hans Kraus, September 24, 1957, PCPF Records.

46. Robert H. Boyle, "The Report that Shocked the President," *Sports Illustrated*, August 15, 1955, 72–73; "Is American Youth Physically Fit?" *U.S. News & World Report*, August 2, 1957, 72.

47. MacCarthy, "Enjoy Keeping Fit."

48. *Fitness in Action*, October 1959, PCPF Records.

49. Untitled clipping, undated (circa summer 1956), *Corpus Christi Caller Times*, Harte File, PCPF Records.

50. Mrs. M. Berger to Carter Burgess, June 3, 1957, PCPF Records.

51. "Special Report," October–November 1960, Council Reports to the Vice President and Memorandums File, PCPF Records.

52. Report on "Recommendations Made at the Second Annual Meeting of the President's Citizens Advisory Committee on the Fitness of American Youth with the President's Council on Youth Fitness and a Summary of Fitness Activities during Fiscal 1959," PCPF Records.

53. *Fitness in Action*, April and August 1960, PCPF Records.

54. Report on meeting of PCYF and PCAC (fiscal 1959), PCPF Records. Reporting back to the PCYF, the chair of the Illinois Governor's Advisory Committee related the events organized in one town: "What happened in Champaign-Urbana may be fairly typical: Two TV presentations, three radio interviews, an editorial in each of two papers, fifteen news stories stressing everything from what was to happen in the elementary schools to what was going on in the YMCA and the Recreation Department. . . . The Junior Olympics, a 'Y' project attracted more than six hundred participants. . . . Over 4,000 young men . . . at the University took a three-item test, chinning, sitting tucks and the mile run. . . . Your chairman had four interviews (TV, Radio and Newspaper) and also opened the week by speaking on 'The Challenge of Fitness' to 150 officers in the area's PTA groups." *Fitness in Action*, June 1959, PCPF Records.

55. Community involvement in fitness was achieved by including members of various nonprofits in the PCAC. For example, representatives from the Jaycees, Amateur Athletic Union, Church of Latter-Day Saints, and Boys' Clubs of America attended the 1958 annual meeting. *Fitness of American Youth: Report of the Second Annual Meeting of the President's Council on Youth Fitness and the President's Citizens Advisory Committee on the Fitness of American Youth* (Washington, D.C.: U.S. Government Printing Office, 1958), 51–55. *Fitness in Action*, the PCYF's newsletter, detailed local and nonprofit fitness programs each month. The June 1959 issue, for example, mentions the establishment of a youth fitness committee for the National Catholic Camping Association; the "activation" of 974 General Federation of Women's Clubs projects involving fitness for youth; the Richmond, Virginia, Jaycees' spon-

sorship of a "road-e-o" for teenagers; and the creation of a Dayton, Ohio, youth fitness committee.

56. "Seventh Monthly Report, April 20, 1958," PCPF Records.

57. *Fitness of American Youth: A Report to the President*, 39–46.

58. William D. Jackson to Shane MacCarthy, August 10, 1959, PCPF Records.

59. Shane MacCarthy to All Council Members, January 20, 1958, PCPF Records; Carl Spielvogel, "Advertising: Wheaties Returns to Sports," *New York Times*, May 21, 1958, 55; "Soaring Bob Richards Sells Physical Fitness to America," *New York Herald Tribune*, August 3, 1958, Special Advertising Section, 4.

60. Bullis was a member of the PCAC in 1958, the year the partnership was solidified. *Fitness of American Youth: Report of the First Annual Conference of the President's Council on Youth Fitness and the President's Citizens Advisory Committee on the Fitness of American Youth* (West Point, N.Y.: U.S. Government Printing Office, 1957), 51, 56. In 1959, Bullis was replaced on the committee by James S. Fish, General Mills's vice president and director of advertising. "Photo News," *Modern Millwheel*, July 1960, 16. On at least one occasion, MacCarthy sent PCYF promotional materials to Knox-Reeves for advice on artwork and layout. Shane MacCarthy to Harry Bullis, December 23, 1958, PCPF Records.

61. Spielvogel, "Advertising: Wheaties Returns to Sports," 55.

62. Fred Biester, Glenbard Township High School, Glen Ellyn, Ill., to Shane MacCarthy, April 24, 1959, PCPF Records.

63. Homer Wadsworth to W. W. Bauer, February 23, 1959, PCPF Records.

64. Bob King to Richard Nixon, July 26, 1955, PCPF Records.

65. Teresa C. Winchell to Floyd Dotson, July 29, 1958, PCPF Records; Eugene Gilbert, *Advertising and Marketing to Young People* (Pleasantville, N.Y.: Printers' Ink, 1957).

66. Tom Englehardt, *The End of Victory Culture: Cold War America and the Disillusioning of a Generation* (New York: Basic Books, 1995), 134; Gilbert, *A Cycle of Outrage*, 196–221.

67. Catherine Reef, *Childhood in America* (New York: Facts on File, 2002), 241–242.

68. Victor Gold, "Crusade for Youth Fitness Invades Host of Outlets," *Public Relations Journal* 17, 1 (1961): 22–24.

69. Robert M. Hoffman, "Telling and Selling the Fitness Story," in President's Council on Youth Fitness, *Recreation Planning for Fitness: Workshop Report No. 8* (Washington, D.C.: U.S. Government Printing Office, 1960), 8–23.

70. Untitled photograph, PCPF Records.

71. Clipping of Safeway grocery store advertisement, *Washington Post*, May 7, 1959, PCPF Records.

72. Carter Burgess to Shane MacCarthy, May 1, 1959, PCPF Records.

73. "Palooka Family Takes to Bowling Lanes," *Bowling World*, undated clipping, PCPF Records. The poster also appeared in the *Cleveland Kegler*, September 9, 1958, 10.

74. John Dell, "There's a Rub in Youth Fitness Drive," *Philadelphia Inquirer*, January 23, 1960, C11.

75. Nan Robertson, "Miss Youth Fitness Puts in a Full Day Exercising," *New York Times*, January 31, 1959, 11.

76. Dell, "There's a Rub in Youth Fitness Drive," C11.

77. Robertson, "Miss Youth Fitness Puts in a Full Day Exercising," 11.

78. *What's My Line?* episode 447, aired January 11, 1959; *To Tell the Truth*, aired February 4, 1960.

79. Dorothy Gilfert, PCYF staff member, to Ethel Dougherty, February 4, 1960, Miss Youth Fitness File, PCPF Records.

80. Irwin Poché, athletic director of the New Orleans Athletic Club, speaking to the New Orleans Public School Athletic League, quoted in *Fitness in Action*, April 1959, PCPF Records.

81. Vincent Bellew to Dwight Eisenhower, undated (circa September 14, 1955), PCPF Records.

82. Dorothy Barclay, "Softness—or Fitness," *New York Times Magazine*, May 13, 1956, 48.

83. "Fitness of American Youth," *Journal of the American Medical Association* 165, 1 (1957): 54–55.

84. Linda K. Kerber, "The Republican Mother: Women and the Enlightenment—An American Perspective," *American Quarterly* 28, 2 (Summer 1976): 187–205.

85. MacCarthy, "Enjoy Keeping Fit," 4–6.

86. Elaine Tyler May, *Homeward Bound: American Families in the Cold War Era* (New York: Basic Books, 1988), 135–149.

87. President's Council on Youth Fitness, *Fitness Can Keep US Strong* (Washington, D.C.: U.S. Government Printing Office, 1960).

88. Shane MacCarthy, "Youth Achieves Fitness through Discipline," address to the University of Kansas School of Medicine, October 6, 1960, transcript, PCPF Records. Media discussions of youth fitness often included mental health issues as well. See, for example, Boyle, "The Report that Shocked the President," 31, 33; Pope, "How Fit Are Our Children?" 92.

89. MacCarthy, "Youth Achieves Fitness through Discipline."

90. President's Council on Youth Fitness, *Guidelines for Physical Evaluation for Youth Fitness* (Washington, D.C.: U.S. Government Printing Office, 1960).

91. Quoted in Mary Louise Adams, *The Trouble with Normal: Postwar Youth and the Making of Heterosexuality* (Toronto: University of Toronto Press, 1997), 92–93.

92. Stephanie Coontz, *The Way We Never Were: American Families and the Nostalgia Trap* (New York: Basic Books, 1992), 25. Although the 1950s were a prosperous time for most white middle-class and many working-class Americans, millions of Americans of color, poor southerners, and those in rural areas were unable to take advantage of the nation's prosperity.

93. Englehardt, *The End of Victory Culture*, 133–134.

94. A number of scholars have explored the significance of this moment. See, for example, May, *Homeward Bound*, 16–18, 162–164; Lizabeth Cohen, *A Consumer's Republic: The Politics of Mass Consumption in Postwar America* (New York: Knopf, 2003), 126; Ruth Feldstein, *Motherhood in Black and White: Race and Sex in American Liberalism, 1930–65* (Ithaca, N.Y.: Cornell University Press, 2000), 114.

95. *Fitness of American Youth: A Report to the President*, 3.

96. See, for example, "What's Wrong with American Youths," 35–36; Pope, "How Fit Are Our Children?" 69; "Are We Becoming Soft?" 35–36; Kelly, "Are We Becoming a Nation of Weaklings?" 26–28.

97. Senator George H. Bender, "Physical Fitness Problem Faces Young America," *This Week in Washington* (constituent newsletter), August 27, 1955, 1, PCPF Records.

98. Paul Boyer, *Promises to Keep: The United States since World War II* (Lexington, Mass.: D. C. Heath, 1995), 127.

99. Englehardt, *The End of Victory Culture*, 149.

100. Lynn Spigel, *Make Room for TV: Television and the Family Ideal in Postwar America* (Chicago: University of Chicago Press, 1992), 50–51.

101. Henderson, "Are We and Our Children Getting Too Soft?" 26–28.

102. Ibid.

103. Spigel, *Make Room for TV*, 52.

104. See, for example, "Is American Youth Physically Fit?" 66–77; Stull, "Conference at Annapolis," 22–24; "Are We Becoming Soft?" 35; Henderson, "Are We and Our Children Getting Too Soft?"; Kelly, "Are We Becoming a Nation of Weaklings?" 26.

105. Quoted in Roberta Park, *Measurement of Physical Fitness: A Historical Perspective* (Washington, D.C.: U.S. Department of Health and Human Services, Public Health Service, 1988), 5.

106. Jarvis, *The Male Body at War*, 19, 61.

107. "Are We Becoming Soft?" 35–36.

108. "What's Wrong with American Youths."

109. Hanson Baldwin, "Our Fighting Men Have Gone Soft," *Saturday Evening Post*, August 8, 1959, 15.

110. Ibid.

111. Ibid., 13.

112. Secretary of Defense's Advisory Committee on Prisoners of War, *POW: The Fight Continues after the Battle* (Washington, D.C.: U.S. Government Printing Office, 1955), 8.

113. Eugene Kinkead, "A Reporter at Large: The Study of Something New in History," *New Yorker*, October 24, 1957, 114. See also Baldwin, "Our Fighting Men Have Gone Soft," 13–15.

114. Kinkead, "A Reporter at Large," 114.

115. Ibid.

116. "A Mean and Cruel Heart," *Time*, August 22, 1955, time.com, accessed September 15, 2011; "G.I. Goes on Trial in 3 Korea Deaths," *New York Times*, August 2, 1955, 5.

117. Kinkead, "A Reporter at Large," 155.

118. Ibid., 157–158.

119. Eugene Kinkead, "The Staff Writer Considers Youth Fitness," in President's Council on Youth Fitness, *Communications Media Forum, Magazine Forum, Broadcasting Forum Workshop Report Nos. 2, 3 and 4* (Washington, D.C.: U.S. Government Printing Office, 1960).

120. Adam J. Zwieback, "The 21 'Turncoat GIs': Nonrepatriations and the Political Culture of the Korean War," *Historian* 60 (Winter 1998): 345–362; Susan L. Carruthers, *Cold War Captives: Imprisonment, Escape and Brainwashing* (Berkeley: University of California Press, 2009), 175.

121. Donald James Adams quoted in David Seed, *Brainwashing: The Fictions of Mind Control* (Kent, Ohio: Kent State University Press, 2004), 27. See Seed's second chapter for a more complete history of the political circulation of this term.

122. "Armed Forces: The Dreadful Dilemma," *Time*, March 22, 1954, time.com, accessed September 15, 2011.

123. Carruthers, *Cold War Captives*, 185.

124. Kinkead, "A Reporter at Large," 118.

125. Virginia Pasley, *21 Stayed: The Story of the American GIs Who Chose Communist China—Who They Were and Why They Stayed* (New York: Farrar, Straus & Cudahy, 1955); Philip Deane, *I Was a Captive in Korea* (New York: Norton, 1953); William L. White, *Captives of Korea: An Unofficial White Paper on the Treatment of War Prisoners: Our Treatment of Theirs, Their Treatment of Ours* (New York: Scribner, 1957); Philip Crosbie, *March til They Die* (Westminster, Md.: Newman Press, 1956); Kenneth K. Hansen, He-

roes behind Barbed Wire (Princeton, N.J.: Van Nostrand, 1957); Edward Hunter, *Brainwashing: The Story of Men Who Defied It* (New York: Farrar, Straus & Cudahy, 1956).

126. David Seed has compiled an extensive list of such books and movies, including *Hold Back the Night* (1952 book), *The Brainwashed Pilot* (1955 film), *A Ride to Panmunjom* (1956 book), *Toward the Unknown* (1956 film), *Sword and Scalpel* (1957 book), *The Rack* (1957 film), and *Night* (1960 book). Seed, *Brainwashing*, 81–105. Susan Carruthers has added to this compilation with NBC's *The Traitor* (1953), MGM's 1954 film *Prisoner of War*, and Columbia Pictures' 1954 *The Bamboo Prison*. Carruthers, *Cold War Captives*, 196–198.

127. Carruthers, *Cold War Captives*, 207.

128. Donald W. Scott, "City Urged to Map Youth Fitness Unit," *Camden (N.J.) Courier-Post*, February 11, 1960, 5.

129. Marjorie Dent Candee, ed., "Carter L. Burgess," in *Current Biography Yearbook* (New York: H. W. Wilson, 1957), 87–89.

130. Kinkead, "A Reporter at Large," 115.

131. Secretary of Defense's Advisory Committee, *POW: The Fight Continues*, 40.

132. Ibid., 31.

133. Ibid., 13.

134. *Fitness of American Youth: Report of the First Annual Conference*, 34.

135. Homer Wadsworth to Shane MacCarthy, November 30, 1959, PCPF Records.

136. President's Council on Youth Fitness, *Fitness Is More than Physical* (Washington, D.C.: U.S. Government Printing Office, 1960).

137. The workshop for religious leaders, which was held February 5, 1960, was one of a series of workshops for various industries that replaced the annual meeting in 1960.

138. President's Council on Youth Fitness, *Religious Group Leaders: Workshop No. 5* (Washington, D.C.: U.S. Government Printing Office, 1960).

139. Marion Hanks, First Council of the 70, Church of Jesus Christ of Latter-Day Saints, to Shane MacCarthy, April 30, 1959, Hanks File, PCPF Records.

140. Marion Hanks to Shane MacCarthy, December 2, 1959, ibid.; see also John Bibby, General Presbyter, United Presbyterian Church, to Theophilus Taylor, Pittsburgh Theological Seminary, February 9, 1960, Religious Workshop File, PCPF Records.

141. Drafts of twenty-second radio spots for Youth Fitness Week, June 1–7, 1958, Fellowes File, PCPF Records.

142. Shane MacCarthy to Edward Greenwood, April 2, 1959, PCPF Records.

143. MacCarthy, "Enjoy Keeping Fit," 4–6.

144. Philip Barba, M.D., University of Pennsylvania Medical School, to Shane MacCarthy, November 20, 1957, PCAC Achievement Guidelines Correspondence File, PCPF Records.

145. Philip Broughton, Mellon Trust, to Shane MacCarthy, June 10, 1959, PCPF Records.

146. John F. Kennedy, "The Soft American," *Sports Illustrated*, December 26, 1960, 15–17.

147. Homer Bigart, "Eisenhower Talk on Fitness Asked," *New York Times*, September 11, 1957, 17; "Kennedy to Push Fitness Program," *New York Times*, December 21, 1960, 22; James Feron, "Fitness of Youths Urged by Kennedy," *New York Times*, July 20, 1961, 1, 14.

148. Dwight Eisenhower to Richard Nixon, July 11, 1955, document 1503, Eisenhower Papers.

149. Donald P. Zingale, "'Ike' Revisited on Sport and National Fitness," *Research Quarterly for Exercise and Sport* 48, 1 (1977): 12–18.

150. In 1957 and 1958, the council's total annual budget was about $140,000, 45 percent of which was funded by the Department of Defense, with other departments contributing 10 to 15 percent each. Minutes of the Internal Advisory Group meeting, July 30, 1957, IAG Meeting Minutes File, PCPF Records; Bigart, "Eisenhower Talk on Fitness Asked," 17.

151. Don Maxwell of Odessa, Texas, writing in the *Sporting Goods Dealer* (a trade publication), January 1959, 144, clipping in PCPF Records.

152. Quoted in Peter Bunzel, "Health Kick's High Priest," *Life*, September 29, 1958, 71–75.

CHAPTER 2. "YOUR HONEYMOON FIGURE"

1. Peter Wyden, *The Overweight Society* (New York: Pocket Books, 1965), vii.

2. Throughout this chapter, I attribute trends of this era to "the 1960s," even though many of them actually emerged in the last years of the 1950s.

3. *Spring thru Summer 1960* (Chicago: Sears Roebuck, 1960), 992; *Spring through Summer 1970* (Chicago: Sears Roebuck, 1970), 313A–313F, 833–835.

4. "Off the Fat of the Land," *Newsweek*, April 20, 1970, 86.

5. For more on federal fitness efforts under Kennedy, see, for example, John F. Kennedy, "The Soft American," *Sports Illustrated*, December 26, 1960, 15–17; "Kennedy to Push Fitness Program," *New York Times*, December 21, 1960, 22; John F. Kennedy, "The Vigor We Need," *Sports Illustrated*, July 16, 1962, 12–14; John F. Kennedy, "Physical Fitness: A Report of Progress," *Look*, August 13, 1963, 82–83.

6. President's Council on Physical Fitness, *Vim: A Complete Exercise Plan for Girls 12 to 18* (Washington, D.C.: U.S. Government Printing Office, 1964); President's Council on Physical Fitness, *Vigor: A Complete Exercise Plan for Boys 12 to 18* (Washington, D.C.: U.S. Government Printing Office, 1964).

7. Victor Gold, "Crusade for Youth Fitness Invades Host of Outlets," *Public Relations Journal* 17, 1 (1961): 22–24.

8. Olga Ley, "Secret Workout," *Redbook*, May 1969, R-2.

9. Bess Furman, "Obesity Is Termed No. 1 Nutritional Ill," *New York Times*, December 9, 1952, 45; "Obesity Is Now No. 1 U.S. Nutritional Problem," *Science News Letter*, December 27, 1952, 408.

10. D. B. Armstrong et al., "Obesity and Its Relation to Health and Disease," *Journal of the American Medical Association* 147 (1951): 1007; Louis I. Dublin, "America's Number One Health Problem," *Today's Health*, September 1952, 18–21; *Build and Blood Pressure Study* (Chicago: Society of Actuaries, 1959); *Obesity and Health* (Arlington, Va.: U.S. Public Health Service, 1966); Roberta Pollack Seid, *Never Too Thin: Why Women Are at War with Their Bodies* (New York: Prentice Hall Press, 1989), 118–124, 139–143; Peter Stearns, *Fat History: Bodies and Beauty in the Modern West*, 2nd ed. (New York: New York University Press, 2002), 109–116.

11. Robert J. Kuczmarski et al., "Prevalence of Overweight among US Adults," *Journal of the American Medical Association* 272, 3 (1994): 205–211.

12. Dublin, "America's Number One Health Problem," 18–21; "34 Million Fatties," *Time*, March 23, 1953, 67; Gerald Walker, "The Great American Dieting Neurosis," *New York Times Magazine*, August 23, 1959, 12, 100; Lawrence Galton, "Why We Are Overly Larded," *New York Times Magazine*, January 15, 1961, 37–50; Jane E. Brody, "Obesity Called a Rising Health Hazard," *New York Times*, July 16, 1966, 1, 23; Stearns, *Fat History*.

13. Stearns, *Fat History*, 130–132.

14. Hillel Schwartz, *Never Satisfied: A Cultural History of Diets, Fantasies and Fat* (New York: Free Press, 1986), 337; Stearns, *Fat History*, 129.

15. Jack Gould, "TV: 'Flabby American,'" *New York Times*, May 31, 1961, 67. The show, which aired on May 30, 1961, and was produced by John Lynch, was part of the network's *Closeup on ABC* series. See also Larry Wolters, "TV Gives a Grim View of 'Flabby American,'" *Chicago Daily Tribune*, May 31, 1961, A4.

16. *CBS Reports: The Fat American*, aired on January 18, 1962. See also Lawrence Laurent, "CBS Is Skating toward 'Thin' Ice," *Washington Post*, January 18, 1962, D8.

17. *Howard K. Smith News and Comment: The Lazy American*, directed by Jack Sameth, aired July 18, 1962, on ABC.

18. "Exercise: A Key to Reducing and Health," *Good Housekeeping*, April 1963, 197. See also Dorothy Stull, "Be Happy, Go Healthy with Bonnie," *Sports Illustrated*, July 16, 1956, 38; Bonnie Prudden, "How to Get More out of Life," *Sports Illustrated*, August 5, 1957, 36; Jean Mayer, "Muscular State of the Union," *New York Times Magazine*, November 6, 1955, 17; Galton, "Why We Are Overly Larded," 47; Marcia Winn, "Why Is Johnny Always Tired?" *Chicago Tribune*, October 20, 1957, G1.

19. Paul Boyer, *Promises to Keep: The United States since World War II* (Lexington, Mass.: D. C. Heath, 1995), 131.

20. Mark S. Foster, *A Nation on Wheels: The Automobile Culture in America since 1945* (Belmont, Calif.: Thomson/Wadsworth, 2003), 53, 58.

21. Ibid., 60.

22. Kenneth T. Jackson, *Crabgrass Frontier: The Suburbanization of the United States* (Oxford: Oxford University Press, 1985), 239.

23. "Flypaper of Suburban Routine," *U.S. News & World Report*, August 2, 1957, 73.

24. Thomas Hine, *Populuxe* (New York: Knopf, 1986), 39, 41, 44.

25. Dorothy Stull, "A Measure of Fitness," *Sports Illustrated*, August 5, 1957, 28–34.

26. Marcia Winn, "Easy Way to More Muscle," *Chicago Daily Tribune*, November 5, 1957, A1.

27. Dorothy Stull, "A Fit Week for a Second Look," *Sports Illustrated*, May 26, 1958, 37–47; John Keats, *Schools without Scholars* (Boston: Houghton Mifflin, 1958), 129–132, 164.

28. Hine, *Populuxe*, 43.

29. Andrew Wiese, *Places of Their Own: African American Suburbanization in the Twentieth Century* (Chicago: University of Chicago Press, 2004), 5.

30. Furman, "Obesity Is Termed No. 1 Nutritional Ill," 45.

31. Jane Stern and Michael Stern, *American Gourmet* (New York: HarperCollins, 1991), x.

32. Ibid., 57–59, 97–110. See also Sylvia Lovegren, *Fashionable Food: Seven Decades of Food Fads* (New York: Macmillan, 1995), 217–267.

33. Stern and Stern, *American Gourmet*, 168–174.

34. Lori Rotskoff, *Love on the Rocks: Men, Women, and Alcohol in Post–World War II America* (Chapel Hill: University of North Carolina Press, 2002), 201–202.

35. Wyden, *The Overweight Society*, 17. See also U.S.D.A. Economics Research Service, "Major Trends in US Food Supply, 1909–1999," *Food Review* 23, 1 (January 2000): 1–15.

36. According to Wyden, beef consumption rose from 148.5 pounds per year in the late 1940s to 170.6 pounds in 1963 (*The Overweight Society*, 10). See also "Pro-

filing Food Consumption in America," www.usda.gov/factbook/chapter2.pdf (accessed February 22, 2012), for a more complete breakdown of meat consumption trends.

37. Galton, "Why We Are Overly Larded," 47, 50. See also Susan Strasser, *Never Done: A History of American Housework*, 2nd ed. (New York: Henry Holt, 2000), 272.

38. Harvey Levenstein, *Paradox of Plenty: A Social History of Eating in Modern America* (New York: Oxford University Press, 1993), 109.

39. Hine, *Populuxe*, 25–26.

40. Daniel Levy and Susan Brink, *A Change of Heart: How the Framingham Heart Study Helped Unravel the Mysteries of Cardiovascular Disease* (New York: Knopf, 2005), 26. American companies produced 320 million pounds of potato chips in 1950 and 532 million pounds in 1960.

41. Lester David, "The Fat Child Can Be Helped," *Good Housekeeping*, February 1962, 124–130.

42. Donna R. Gabaccia, *We Are What We Eat: Ethnic Food and the Making of Americans* (Cambridge, Mass.: Harvard University Press, 1998), 165.

43. Richard Pillsbury, *No Foreign Food: The American Diet in Time and Place* (Boulder, Colo.: Westview Press, 1998), 72–73, 182–183.

44. Wyden, *The Overweight Society*, 18.

45. Ibid., 17.

46. Stanley Garn, "Growth and Development," in *Our Nation's Children*, ed. Eli Ginzberg (New York: Columbia University Press, 1960), 35; "Nation's Youth Getting Too Fat, Report for White House Finds," *New York Times*, March 1, 1960, 35.

47. Seid, *Never Too Thin*, 136.

48. Ibid., 109.

49. Levenstein, *Paradox of Plenty*, 136.

50. Seid, *Never Too Thin*, 109–111.

51. Karal Ann Marling, *As Seen on TV: The Visual Culture of Everyday Life in the 1950s* (Cambridge, Mass.: Harvard University Press, 1996), 43.

52. Lois Banner, *American Beauty* (Chicago: University of Chicago Press, 1983), 283–290.

53. Dorris Conway, "Our Fat Children," *Ladies' Home Journal*, April 1961, 14–19.

54. Jean Noe, "New Fashions Stress the Unfettered Body," *Virgin Islands Daily News*, January 17, 1966, 5.

55. Kathy Peiss, *Hope in a Jar: The Making of America's Beauty Culture* (New York: Metropolitan Books, 1998), 203–237; Carolyn de la Pena, *Empty Pleasures: The Story of Artificial Sweeteners from Saccharin to Splenda* (Chapel Hill: University of North Carolina Press, 2010), 41–42.

56. Stearns, *Fat History*, 89–93.

57. Era Bell Thompson, "How to Lose Weight without Half Trying," *Ebony*, June 1968, 123–130.

58. Fashion models Naomi Sims and Donyale Luna had begun to appear on magazine covers in Europe and the United States by the late 1960s.

59. For more about California culture in the 1960s, see Kirse Granat May, *Golden State, Golden Youth: The California Image in Popular Culture, 1955–1966* (Chapel Hill: University of North Carolina Press, 2002).

60. *Gidget*, directed by Paul Wendkos, Columbia Pictures, 1959; *Gidget Goes Hawaiian*, directed by Paul Wendkos, Columbia Pictures, 1961; *Gidget*, ABC, 1965–1966.

61. *Muscle Beach Party*, directed by William Asher, American International Pictures, 1964; *How to Stuff a Wild Bikini*, directed by William Asher, American International Pictures, 1965.

62. "California Beauty Wherever You Live," *Good Housekeeping*, January 1963, 70–71; "California Woman," *Ladies' Home Journal*, July 1967, 61–63.

63. Campaigns that emphasized an active lifestyle began as early as 1966. Specific activities were featured in 1968 and 1969. See, for example, "Run. Whirl. Roar. Have Fun," *Good Housekeeping*, May 1966, 27. Cutex nail polish also ran a campaign entitled "Catch a Perfect Wave of Color" that featured surfboard-riding models; see, for example, *Redbook*, July 1967, 9.

64. Gael Greene, "For the Single Girl: A New Way of Life in California," *Ladies' Home Journal*, July 1966, 58–59, 110–112.

65. See, for example, "Salt-Water Notes for a Sportsman's Biography," *Sports Illustrated*, December 26, 1960, 23; James Feron, "Fitness of Youths Urged by Kennedy," *New York Times*, July 20, 1961, 1, 14; "The President Who Loved Sports," *Sports Illustrated*, December 2, 1963, 20–21.

66. "One! Two! Up! Down! Push! Tug! Twist! Touch! Bend! Stretch!" *Gentlemen's Quarterly*, February 1964, 102–103.

67. Susan J. Douglas, *Where the Girls Are: Growing up Female with the Mass Media* (New York: Random House, 1994), 39.

68. Dawn Crowell Ney, "I Lost 145 Pounds," *Ladies' Home Journal*, March 1962, 18; E. S. Hughes, "How I Lost Eighty Pounds in 19 Weeks," *Ladies' Home Journal*, October 1968, 83; Dawn Crowell Ney, "Too Pretty to Be Fat," *Ladies' Home Journal*, January 1962, 10; Dawn Crowell Ney, "Pretty but Fat," *Ladies' Home Journal*, October 1961, 49; "My Husband Deserved Better," *Good Housekeeping*, April 1968, 70–74.

69. Walker, "The Great American Dieting Neurosis," 12; Seid, *Never Too Thin*, 105.

70. Bonnie Prudden, *How to Keep Slender and Fit after Thirty* (New York: Random House, 1961), 61.

71. Harriet Van Horne, "If You're on a Diet, Shut Up!" *Redbook*, September 1968, 58–60.

72. "Wise Woman's Diet for Summer Slimming," *Redbook*, July 1967, 84–87.

73. Stanley Frank, "Illusions of Reducing," *Saturday Evening Post*, January 20, 1962, 28–31.

74. *Spring through Summer 1960*, 1001.

75. Advertisement for Correctol, "Dieting to Reduce?" *Ladies' Home Journal*, May 1961, 37.

76. Schwartz, *Never Satisfied*, 204. See also "34 Million Fatties," 67.

77. "Shape up and Slim Down (with 68 Diet Tips and Eight Lazy Exercises)," *Good Housekeeping*, January 1967, 154–158.

78. Wallace Croatman, "How to Stay Well in the Winter," *Redbook*, February 1960, 24.

79. Jean Nidetch, "Ask Jean Nidetch," *Weight Watchers Magazine*, February 1968, 4–6.

80. Ruth Brecker and Edward Brecker, "All about Diets," *Redbook*, March 1960, 38–39, 79–84. See also "34 Million Fatties," 67; "Exercise—What It's Doing for Ike and What It Can Do for You," *U.S. News & World Report*, August 23, 1957, 50–59.

81. Walter E. O'Donnell, "A Doctor Talks Sense about Diet," *Good Housekeeping*, October 1966, 260–266.

82. E. Philip Gelvin and Thomas H. McGavack, *Obesity: Its Cause, Classification and Care* (New York: Hoeber-Harper, 1957), 73.

83. Seymour Halpern, "What Too Many Women Don't Know about Dieting," *Redbook*, September 1969, 82–87.

84. Jean Mayer, "Exercise Does Keep the Weight Down," *Atlantic*, July 1955, 63–66; Mayer, "Muscular State of the Union," 17; Dorothy Stull, "What to Do after a Heart Attack? Exercise!" *Sports Illustrated*, January 2, 1956, 44–47; "Exercise—What It's Doing for Ike," 50–59.

85. See, for example, the exercises demonstrated in *Good Housekeeping's Plan for Reducing* (Columbia Records, 1960); *Harper's Bazaar's Secret Formula for a Beautiful New You* (Capitol Records, 1961); Debbie Drake, *Feel Good! Look Great! Exercise along with Debbie Drake* (Epic Records LM 26034, 1963); Ed Allen, *Ed Allen Time* (Ed Allen Enterprises, circa 1965).

86. "Shape up for Summer," *Good Housekeeping*, May 1969, 132–136; "Everybody into the Water," *Redbook*, June 1969, 82–87.

87. Ley, "Secret Workout," R-2.

88. "Body Rhythms," *Good Housekeeping*, January 1962, 71–74; "TV's Nature Boy," *Look*, August 30, 1960, 28–30.

89. "Shape up for Summer," 132–136.

90. "How Effective Are Those 'No Work' Exercise Devices?" *Good Housekeeping*, August 1970, 145–147; "Off the Fat of the Land," 86, 91. See also retail catalogs of the era, which mingle electronic stimulation devices with barbells and treadmills.

91. Debbie Drake, *How to Keep Your Husband Happy. Look Slim! Keep Trim! Exercise along with Debbie Drake* (Epic Records BN 26102, 1964).

92. Ibid.

93. Ibid.

94. Prudden, *How to Keep Slender and Fit after Thirty*, 208.

95. "Sego Liquid Diet Formula," *Ladies' Home Journal*, July–August 1963, 25.

96. "Verve Transistor Relax-a-Cizor," *Good Housekeeping*, January 1960, 131.

97. Farley Heward, "I Lost My Husband before I Lost 70 Pounds," *Ladies' Home Journal*, October 1967, 33.

98. Marsha F. Cassidy, *What Women Watched: Daytime Television in the 1950s* (Austin: University of Texas Press, 2005), 7–8.

99. A handful of episodes of *The Jack La Lanne Show* made their way to the UCLA Film and Television Archive. The most complete collection is held by La Lanne's company BeFit Enterprises, which continues to use them for profit through television advertising and DVD sales. Episodes packaged for resale are not dated beyond the year of production, if at all. For a brief period in 2005, cable channel ESPN Classic broadcast the show; although the original airdates were not specified, the shows were clearly from La Lanne's early period (1958–1962), as evidenced by his requests that viewers recommend the new program to their friends to ensure that it stayed on the air.

100. Cassidy, *What Women Watched*, 8–11.

101. John Cassidy, "Still Pumped Up," *New Yorker*, November 25, 2002.

102. La Lanne's opening credits typically depicted him in silhouette doing jumping jacks. Although some contemporary sources claim that La Lanne invented the jumping jack, La Lanne's early shows treated it like any other exercise.

103. "Exercise Break?" *Christian Science Monitor*, July 8, 1965, 14.

104. "Helpmate for Herenow," *Newsweek*, July 25, 1960, 102.

105. Jack La Lanne, *The Jack La Lanne Way to Vibrant Good Health* (New York: Prentice-Hall, 1960), 45–48.

106. "One & Kick & Two, and Stick out Your Tongue," *Time*, February 16, 1968, 52.

107. *The Jack La Lanne Show*, aired on ESPN Classic January 11, 2005 (original airdate unavailable).

108. *The Jack La Lanne Show*, aired on ESPN Classic January 20, 2005 (original airdate unavailable).

109. "TV's Nature Boy," 28–30.

110. Cassidy, *What Women Watched*, 76, 100.

111. Huston Horn, "La Lanne: A Treat and a Treatment," *Sports Illustrated*, December 19, 1960, 28–31.

112. Tim Kiska, *From Soupy to Nuts! A History of Detroit Television* (Royal Oak, Mich.: Monumentum, 2005), 25–26.

113. "Letters to Louise," *Chicago Tribune*, March 18, 1963, B11.

114. "One & Kick & Two," 52; James Ritch, "Ed Allen, 55 Pushups and Me," *Chicago Tribune*, August 5, 1961, A3.

115. "The Locust, the Lotus, the Plough, the Cobra," *TV Guide*, February 10, 1962, 10–12.

116. Ibid.

117. Larry Wolters, "Mr. Keep Fit's Back, Ladies, over WGN-TV," *Chicago Daily Tribune*, October 2, 1950, B10. There was also a tie-in book: Paul Fogarty, *Your Figure, Ladies* (New York: A. S. Barnes, 1955).

118. Larry Wolters, "Views Morning Video and Finds Exciting Shows," *Chicago Daily Tribune*, February 28, 1951, A6; Eleanor Nangle, "Chicagoland Women Learn to Streamline Figures," *Chicago Tribune*, May 21, 1951, B1; Larry Wolters, "Exercising Show Has Loyal Fans," *Chicago Tribune*, April 22, 1954, C4.

119. Martha Overholser, "Be Figure Wise, Pound Foolish—See Terry on TV," *Chicago Daily Tribune*, May 3, 1953, SW22.

120. "Debbie Drake, Body Beautifier," *Saturday Evening Post*, November 25, 1961, 29.

121. Drake, *Feel Good! Look Great! Exercise along with Debbie Drake*; Drake, *How to Keep Your Husband Happy. Look Slim! Keep Trim! Exercise along with Debbie Drake*; Debbie Drake, *Debbie Drake's Easy Way to a Perfect Figure and Glowing Health* (Englewood Cliffs, N.J.: Prentice-Hall, 1961); Debbie Drake, *Debbie Drake's Secrets of Perfect Figure Development* (Englewood Cliffs, N.J.: Prentice-Hall, 1965); Debbie Drake, *Dancercize* (Englewood Cliffs, N.J.: Prentice-Hall, 1967).

122. Cindy Sabulis, *Collector's Guide to Dolls of the 1960s and 1970s: Identification and Values*, vol. 1 (Paducah, Ky.: Collector Books, 2000), 142.

123. See, for example, "One, Two," *Time*, May 5, 1961, 52; "Debbie Drake, Body Beautifier," 29.

124. "Letters to Louise," *Chicago Tribune*, March 6, 1963, A1.

125. Cecil Smith, "Exercised Fans Flex Their Pens," *Los Angeles Times*, April 19, 1961, A16.

126. "One, Two."

127. "Lost: 200,000 Pounds," *TV Guide*, November 6, 1954, A2.

128. Ibid., A2, A3; "Personality . . . No. 58," *Pittsburgh Press*, February 21, 1954, clipping from the collection of John Firth.

129. Gloria Roeder, *Exercise with Gloria and Her Six Daughters for Family Fitness Fun* (Exercise with Gloria 6666, 1962).

130. Joan Cook, "Physical Fitness of Youth Has Expert Fit to Be Tied," *New York Times*, May 7, 1959, 40; Stull, "A Fit Week for a Second Look," 37–47.

131. Mrs. Glenn Corbin, Woodland Hills, Calif., to the "Producers of 'It's Fun to Reduce,'" January 8, 1959, in the private collection of John Firth.

132. "Exercise," *Ladies' Home Journal*, November 1965, 94–95.

133. "How to Find More Energy!" *Good Housekeeping*, May 1960, 21.

134. Sara M. Evans, *Born for Liberty: A History of Women in America* (New York: Macmillan, 1989), 251.

135. Cassidy, *What Women Watched*, 118, 194.

136. Maryhelen Vannier, *A Better Figure for You through Easy Exercise and Diet* (New York: Association Press, 1965), 10.

137. Sophia Delza, *Feel Fine, Look Lovely* (New York: Hawthorn, 1969), 14.

138. Quoted in Wyden, *The Overweight Society*, 86.

139. *The Jack La Lanne Show*, aired on ESPN Classic January 25, 2005 (original airdate unavailable).

140. Jack La Lanne, *Abundant Health and Vitality after 40* (Englewood Cliffs, N.J.: Prentice-Hall, 1962), 78.

141. Betty Friedan, *The Feminine Mystique* (New York: Norton, 1963).

CHAPTER 3. THE HEART OF THE MAN IN THE GRAY FLANNEL SUIT

1. "Mr. Wilson's Uncle," *Dennis the Menace*, directed by Charles Barton, aired February 18, 1962.

2. William G. Rothstein, *Public Health and the Risk Factor: A History of an Uneven Medical Revolution* (Rochester, N.Y.: University of Rochester Press, 2003), 1–5.

3. Arthur Blumenfeld, *Heart Attack: Are You a Candidate?* (New York: Paul S. Eriksson, 1964), 7.

4. See, for example, Jesse Stuart, *The Year of My Rebirth* (New York: McGraw-Hill, 1958); Cameron Hawley, *The Hurricane Years* (Boston: Little Brown, 1968); Tex Maule, *Running Scared: The Odyssey of a Heart-Attack Victim's Jogging Back to Health* (New York: Saturday Review Press, 1972). In the 1964 film *Send Me No Flowers* (directed by Norman Jewison, Universal Studios), Rock Hudson plays a hypochondriac in a send-up of the decade's male health concerns.

5. Carleton B. Chapman, "Introduction," in *Prescription for Life*, ed. M. F. Graham (New York: David McKay, 1966), xvii.

6. Todd Olszewski, "Cholesterol: A Scientific, Medical and Social History, 1908–1962" (Ph.D. diss., Yale University, 2008), 69; Paul D. White, *My Life and Medicine: An Autobiographical Memoir* (Boston: Gambit, 1971), 72; Thomas Royle Dawber, *The Framingham Study: The Epidemiology of Atherosclerotic Disease* (Cambridge, Mass.: Harvard University Press, 1980), 11–12; Rothstein, *Public Health and the Risk Factor*, 203.

7. Howard Rusk, "The State of the Union's Health," *New York Times Magazine*, July 22, 1956, 18.

8. Rothstein, *Public Health and the Risk Factor*, 192–195; Maurice Cambell, "The Mortality Rate from Heart Disease," *American Heart Journal* 68, 1 (1964): 1–2; Norman Jolliffe, Seymour Rinzler, and Morton Archer, "The Anti-Coronary Club; Including a Discussion of the Effects of a Prudent Diet on the Serum Cholesterol Level of Middle-Aged Men," *American Journal of Clinical Nutrition* 7 (July–August 1959): 451–462.

9. Jolliffe, Rinzler, and Archer, "The Anti-Coronary Club."

10. William F. Enos, James C. Beyer, and Robert H. Holmes, "Pathogenesis of Coronary Disease in American Soldiers Killed in Korea," *Journal of the American Medical Association* 158, 11 (1955): 912–914; William F. Enos, Robert H. Holmes, and James C. Beyer, "Coronary Disease among United States Soldiers Killed in Action in Korea," *Journal of the American Medical Association* 152 (1953): 1090–1093.

11. Olszewski, "Cholesterol," 103–112; Daniel Steinberg, *The Cholesterol Wars: The Skeptics vs. the Preponderance of Evidence* (San Diego: Elsevier, 2007), 33–35.

12. J. A. Heady, J. N. Morris, and P. A. Raffle, "The Physique of London Busmen: The Epidemiology of Uniforms," *Lancet* 271, 6942 (September 15, 1956): 569–570; J. N. Morris, J. A. Heady, P. A. B. Raffle, C. G. Roberts, and J. W. Parks, "Coronary Heart Disease and Physical Activity of Work," *Lancet* 2 (1953): 1052–1057, 1111–1120.

13. Cary L. Cooper and Philip Dewe, *Stress: A Brief History* (Malden, Mass.: Blackwell, 2004), 14–20.

14. The midcentury notion of men in crisis was advanced, in large part, by sociologists such as C. Wright Mills and William Whyte. Michael Kimmel, *Manhood in America: A Cultural History* (New York: Free Press, 1996), 241–258. For an alternative analysis of the "male panic," see James Gilbert, *Men in the Middle: Searching for Masculinity in the 1950s* (Chicago: University of Chicago Press, 2005).

15. William Attwood and George B. Leonard Jr., *The Decline of the American Male* (New York: Random House, 1958).

16. Barbara Ehrenreich, *The Hearts of Men: American Dreams and the Flight from Commitment* (Garden City, N.Y.: Anchor Press, 1983), 68–87.

17. Hans Selye, *The Stress of Life* (New York: McGraw-Hill, 1956).

18. "Rising Pressures to Perform," *Time*, July 18, 1969, 75.

19. Attwood and Leonard, *Decline of the American Male*.

20. "Rising Pressures to Perform," 75.

21. American Management Association, "The Man in Management: A Personal View Including a Section on Executive Health Problems," *General Management Series* 189 (1957); William Whyte, *The Organization Man* (New York: Simon & Schuster, 1956).

22. "Science Notes: Medicine Focuses on the Care of the American Executive," *New York Times*, April 26, 1959, E9; Howard A. Rusk, "Executives' Health: Physicians at Parley Urge Check-ups and Taking Advice of Satchel Paige," *New York Times*, May 14, 1961, 85.

23. For accounts of the rise of the field of executive health, see George M. Saunders, "Survey of Executive Health Programs," *Archives of Industrial Hygiene and Occupational Medicine* 9, 2 (1954): 133–141; Charles L. Huston, "Management's Responsibility for Executive Health: A Corporate Program," *General Management Series* 189 (1957): 33–42; Charles E. Thompson, Earl A. Zaus, and Philip R. Zeller, "Some Observations on Periodic Executive Health Examinations," *Journal of Occupational Medicine* 3, 4 (April 1961): 215–217; W. P. Shepard, "Executive Health: How to Maintain It," *Archives of Environmental Health* 6 (1963): 312–314; H. A. Vonachen and William J. Roche Jr., "Comparative Study of Executive Health Examinations," *Journal of Occupational Medicine* 5, 8 (1963): 389–394; Harry J. Johnson, "Fifty Years Experience with Executive Health Examinations," *Journal of Occupational Medicine* 9, 6 (1967): 299–303.

24. William Brams, *Managing Your Coronary* (Philadelphia: Lippincott, 1953), 15.

25. Alton Blakeslee and Jeremiah Stamler, *Your Heart Has Nine Lives* (New York: Pocket Books, 1963), 7.

26. Jane Lincoln, "I'm to Blame that My Husband Died Too Young," *Cosmopolitan*, August 1954, 84–89.

27. Hannah Lees, "Our Men Are Killing Themselves," *Saturday Evening Post*, January 28, 1956, 25, 111, 114.

28. Lincoln, "I'm to Blame that My Husband Died Too Young," 84–89.

29. Saunders, "Survey of Executive Health Programs," 133–141.

30. Charles Edward Thompson, *What an Executive Should Know about His Health* (Chicago: Dartnell Corporation, 1961), 14.

31. Quoted in Rothstein, *Public Health and the Risk Factor*, 208.

32. Quoted in Warren R. Guild, *After Your Heart Attack* (New York: Harper & Row, 1969), 75–76.

33. Rothstein, *Public Health and the Risk Factor*, 205–208.

34. See, for example, "They Ran the Heart Study," *Business Week*, December 12, 1964, 51–58; "Coronary Candidates," *Newsweek*, November 4, 1963, 63.

35. Richard E. Lee and Ralph F. Schneider, "Hypertension and Arteriosclerosis in Executive and Nonexecutive Personnel," *Journal of the American Medical Association* 167, 12 (1958): 1447–1450; Richard D. Lyons, "Study Finds Stresses of Success No Peril to Heart," *New York Times*, April 2, 1968, 38; Aaron Antonovsky, "Social Class and the Major Cardiovascular Diseases," *Journal of Chronic Diseases* 21 (1968): 65–106. Antonovsky's article describes the findings in fifty-six studies of heart disease and concludes that the perception that heart disease is related to occupational status is unfounded.

36. Harvey Green, *Fit for America: Health, Fitness, Sport and American Society* (Baltimore: Johns Hopkins University Press, 1988), 137–140. More recently, David Schuster has shown that neurasthenia was diagnosed among immigrants and people of color as the affliction became more widespread. David Schuster, *Neurasthenic Nation: America's Search for Health, Happiness and Comfort, 1869–1920* (New Brunswick, N.J.: Rutgers University Press, 2011), 62–63.

37. Rothstein, *Public Health and the Risk Factor*, 203–205.

38. "Negroes Have One-Fifth Coronary Thrombosis Cases as Whites," *Milwaukee Defender*, March 14, 1957.

39. "Ten Year Study of Blood Vessels of Two Groups Yields Interesting Results," *Baltimore Afro-American*, October 29, 1966, 20.

40. Lees, "Our Men Are Killing Themselves," 25.

41. Olszewski, "Cholesterol," 181.

42. Ibid., 180–181.

43. Jean Libman Block, "How Can I Help My Husband Avoid a Heart Attack," *Reader's Digest*, September 1962, 69–72.

44. Blakeslee and Stamler, *Your Heart Has Nine Lives*, 215.

45. Kenneth C. Hutchin, *How Not to Kill Your Husband* (New York: Hawthorn Books, 1962), 20–21.

46. White, *My Life and Medicine*, 214.

47. Dorothy Stull, "What to Do after a Heart Attack? Exercise!" *Sports Illustrated*, January 2, 1956, 44–47; "Exercise—What It's Doing for Ike and What It Can Do for You," *U.S. News & World Report*, August 23, 1957, 50–59; "How the President Keeps Himself Healthy," *U.S. News & World Report*, August 23, 1957, 60–62; Eugene B. Mozes, *Living beyond Your Heart Attack* (Englewood Cliffs, N.J.: Prentice-Hall, 1959), 83.

48. White, *My Life and Medicine*, 217–218; "Heart Meeting Draws 10,400," *Oregonian*, November 7, 1964, 13; "Dr. Paul Dudley White Schedules Lecture 'Hearts and Husbands,'" *Oregonian*, November 5, 1964, 38; "78-Year Old Cardiologist Maintains Busy Schedule," *Oregonian*, November 6, 1964, 18; "Hearts and Husbands Day," *Deseret (Utah) News*, June 13, 1967, 10B; Paul D. White, "Women Can Help Prevent Tragedy of Needless Heart Disease Deaths," *Modesto (Calif.) Bee*, February 15, 1966, B4; "Application for Tickets," *Wisconsin State Journal*, September 24, 1965, 2–5.

49. "American Wife," circa 1967, Lawrence F. Karr Public Service Announcement Collection, Motion Pictures, Library of Congress.

50. The notion of the wife keeping the dangers and stresses of the outside world from the haven of the home dates from the nineteenth century. See Nancy Wolloch, *Women and the American Experience* (New York: Knopf, 1984), 116–117.

51. Block, "How Can I Help My Husband Avoid a Heart Attack," 69–71.

52. According to Sonneborn, alcohol in moderation posed no risk to heart attack victims. Robert M. Sonneborn, *If Your Husband Has Coronary Heart Disease* (New York: Carlton Press, 1968), 42.

53. "What Was the Date of Your Husband's Last Physical Checkup?" *Ladies' Home Journal*, January 1966, 47.

54. "Will a Beautyrest Help Your Husband Protect His Heart?" *Good Housekeeping*, November 1963, 68–69; "Is One-Third of His Life Worth Anything to You?" *Good Housekeeping*, April 1963, 44–45.

55. "What Wives Should Know about Male Support," *Good Housekeeping*, May 1963, 237.

56. Roberta Pollack Seid, *Never Too Thin: Why Women Are at War with Their Bodies* (New York: Prentice Hall Press, 1989), 115–116.

57. Tom Burke, "Fat and the Single Boy," *Gentlemen's Quarterly*, February 1964, 100–101.

58. Lynne Luciano, *Looking Good: Male Body Image in America* (New York: Hill & Wang, 2001), 81.

59. Olszewski, "Cholesterol," 190.

60. Seid, *Never Too Thin*, 152. Accounts of men's dieting did circulate in popular culture, but they were noteworthy precisely because they were exceptions to the rule. See Jesse Berrett, "Feeding the Organization Man: Diet and Masculinity in Postwar America," *Journal of Social History* 30, 4 (Summer 1997): 805–825.

61. "The New Man," *Gentlemen's Quarterly*, March 1964, 46–49.

62. "Ten Years of Grooming," *Gentlemen's Quarterly*, Winter 1967, 126–127.

63. Dominique Padurano, "Making American Men: Charles Atlas and the Business of Bodies, 1892–1945" (Ph.D. diss., Rutgers University, 2007), 211.

64. F. Valentine Hooven, *Beefcake: The Muscle Magazines of America*, 1950–1970 (Berlin: Taschen Verlag, 1996), 61–64. For additional image comparisons, see David L. Chapman and Brett Josef Grubisic, *American Hunks: The Muscular Male Body in American Culture* (Vancouver: Arsenal Pulp Press, 2009).

65. Untitled drawing, *Playboy*, August 1966, 167, cited in Padurano, "Making American Men."

66. Huston Horn, "La Lanne: A Treat and a Treatment," *Sports Illustrated*, December 19, 1960, 28–31.

67. "Suck in that Gut, America!" *Esquire*, November 1962, 82–85.

68. Robert L. Griswold, *Fatherhood in America: A History* (New York: Basic Books, 1993), 186–198.

69. "Amazing New Way to Reduce the Size of your Waistline," *Gentlemen's Quarterly*, October 1963, 157.

70. Bonnie Prudden, *Executive Fitness* (Warner Bros. Records W 1619, 1965).

71. "If You Want to Stay Healthy . . . ," *Nation's Business*, February 1969, 56–58.

72. Thompson, *What an Executive Should Know about His Health*, 117–119.

73. Harry J. Johnson, *Keeping Fit in Your Executive Job* (New York: American Management Association, 1962), 63–65.

74. See, for example, Phyllis Wright, "Medicine Today," *Ladies' Home Journal*, October 1966, 25.

75. "Latest on Exercise and What It Does for You," *U.S. News & World Report*, June 8, 1959, 104–105.

76. Stull, "What to Do after a Heart Attack?" 44–47. This warning also held true for recommended activities such as golf and tennis. See, for example, "Personal Business," *Business Week*, December 16, 1961, 121.

77. Hutchin, *How Not to Kill Your Husband*, 123; Block, "How Can I Help My Husband Avoid a Heart Attack," 69–71.

78. "Exercise—What It's Doing for Ike," 50–59; "One! Two! Up! Down! Push! Tug! Twist! Touch! Bend! Stretch!" *Gentlemen's Quarterly*, February 1964, 102–103; Curtis Mitchell, "Tennis, Everyone? Or Swimming, or—?" *New York Times Magazine*, April 23, 1961, 57–64; "Personal Business," *Business Week*, January 6, 1968, 95–96.

79. Prudden, *Executive Fitness*; "Personal Business," 95–96.

80. Peter J. Steincrohn, *How to Be Lazy, Healthy and Fit* (New York: Funk & Wagnalls, 1968), 8. Steincrohn's tirade against exercise had begun much earlier; see Peter J. Steincrohn, *You Don't Have to Exercise!* (Garden City, N.Y.: Doubleday, Doran, 1942); Peter J. Steincrohn, *How to Keep Fit without Exercise* (New York: W. Funk, 1952); Peter J. Steincrohn, *Mr. Executive: Keep Well—Live Longer* (New York: Frederick Fell, 1960), 73–82.

81. For examples of the works Steincrohn hoped to counter, see Bonnie Prudden, *How to Keep Slender and Fit after Thirty* (New York: Random House, 1961); Jack La Lanne, *Abundant Health and Vitality after 40* (Englewood Cliffs, N.J.: Prentice-Hall, 1962).

82. Steincrohn, *How to Be Lazy, Healthy and Fit*, 32.

83. Ibid., 9.

84. Ibid., frontispiece. My own copy of Steincrohn's book bears an inscription to another reader in faded ballpoint: "You will like this book. I sure did."

85. Peter Wyden, *The Overweight Society* (New York: Pocket Books, 1965), 98–99.

86. Steincrohn, *How to Be Lazy, Healthy and Fit*, 19.

87. Thomas Cureton Jr., *Physical Fitness and Dynamic Health* (New York: Dial Press, 1965). Cureton's clinics appear to have been sponsored by individual YMCAs. See Phil Casey, "Most of Us Are Middle Aged at 26 and Become 'Lively Fossils' at 40," *Washington Post*, October 30, 1960, B1. For more on Cureton, see Jack W. Berryman, "Thomas K. Cureton, Jr.: Pioneer Researcher, Proselytizer, and Proponent for Physical Fitness," *Research Quarterly for Exercise and Sport* 67, 1 (1996): 1–12.

88. Demographic information on BMCs and their membership was collected in 1946 by YMCA National Council staffer Harold Friermood for his dissertation. See Harold T. Friermood, "Health Clubs in the YMCA with Respect to Current Status and Development of Operating Standards" (Ed.D. diss., New York University, 1954), 19, 58–61, 100–103.

89. Ibid., 140–159.

90. William W. Waxman, "Physical Fitness Developments for Adults in the YMCA," in *Exercise and Fitness: A Collection of Papers Presented at the Colloquium on Exercise and Fitness* (Monticello, Ill.: Athletic Institute, 1959), 183–192.

91. Curtis Mitchell, "New Cure for Sick Hearts," *True*, December 1962, 66–70, 114–115.

92. Ibid.

93. "Measured Mile Program," in Clipping File, Records of the Minneapolis YMCA, Kautz Family YMCA Archives, Minneapolis, Minn. See also "To Kickoff Measured Mile Program Saturday," *Owosso (Mich.) Argus-Press*, May 14, 1963, 3; "For More Walks," *Schenectady (N.Y.) Gazette*, June 11, 1963, 18; "We Salute Measured Mile," *Prescott (Ariz.) Gazette*, September 22, 1974, 2; "YMCA Measured Mile Program for Walkers Scheduled in Glendale," *Los Angeles Times*, April 14, 1963, GB5.

94. Several studies as well as physicians' reports have documented this tendency. See, for example, U.S. Department of Health and Human Services, *Utilization of Ambulatory Medical Care by Women: United States, 1997–98*, Series Report 13, no. 149, July 2001, available at www.cdc.gov/nchs/data/series/sr_13/sr13_149.pdf;

David Sandman, Elisabeth Simantov, and Christina An, *Out of Touch: American Men and the Health Care System* (New York: Commonwealth Fund, 2000).

95. Office of Minority Health, Department of Health and Human Services, "Heart Disease and African Americans," http://minorityhealth.hhs.gov/templates/content.aspx?ID=3018, accessed August 15, 2012.

CHAPTER 4. RUN FOR YOUR LIFE

1. Laurel Shackelford, "Joggers Reach National Status," *Washington Post*, September 24, 1968, B2; "Udall Paces Bipartisan Band of Joggers as National Association Is Born," *New York Times*, September 24, 1968, 34.

2. See, for example, Andrew J. Edelstein and Kevin McDonough, *The Seventies: From Hot Pants to Hot Tubs* (New York: Dutton, 1990), 125–127; David Frum, *How We Got Here: The 70s—The Decade that Brought You Modern Life (for Better or Worse)* (New York: Basic Books, 2000), 173–174; Thomas Borstelmann, *The 1970s: A New Global History from Civil Rights to Economic Inequality* (Princeton, N.J.: Princeton University Press, 2012), 64–70.

3. A similar chronology has also been outlined in Darcy Plymire, "A Moral Exercise: Long Distance Running in the 1970s" (Ph.D. diss., University of Iowa, 1996).

4. Hal Higdon, "Jogging Is an In Sport," *New York Times Magazine*, April 14, 1968, 36; "Agility Counts, Too," *Road and Track*, July 1978, 1, 25.

5. In the earliest years of the movement, *jogging* could denote periods of slow running interspersed with walking until a runner was able to jog continuously. Over the course of the 1970s, *running*— always the preferred term among those with track and field backgrounds—gradually replaced *jogging*. Some joggers/runners have argued that the two terms convey a difference in speed. See, for example, Sidney Landau, "What Do People Call You?" *Runner's World*, January 1975, 28–31; Hal Higdon, "Proud to Be a Jogger," *Runner's World*, December 1976, 29–31. This distinction did not apply to distance, however. The American Medical Joggers Association, for example, recommended marathon running as the best activity to prevent heart disease. For language variety, this chapter uses both terms interchangeably.

6. I borrow the Rorschach test analogy from Hal Higdon, who used it to refer to the Bible in another context. Hal Higdon, "Is Running a Religious Experience?" *Runner's World*, May 1978, 75–79.

7. Lafayette Smith, "Run for Your Health," *Today's Health*, October 1964, 34–37; William J. Bowerman and W. E. Harris, *Jogging: A Physical Fitness Program for All Ages* (New York: Grosset & Dunlap, 1967), 47–55; Kenny Moore, *Bowerman and the Men of Oregon: The Story of Oregon's Legendary Coach and Nike's Cofounder* (Emmaus, Pa.:

Rodale, 2006), 146–155; Thor Gotaas, *Running: A Global History* (London: Reaktion Books, 2009), 240–244; William H. Freeman, "Bill Bowerman: Catalyst of the Jogging Movement," *Sport History Review* 5, 1 (1974): 47–55.

8. "Jog Way to Physical Fitness in Middle Age," *Chicago Tribune*, August 15, 1964, C4; "Top Track Coach Thinks Jogging Ideal as Exercise for Older Men," *Washington Post*, August 15, 1965, C3; Smith, "Run for Your Health," 34–37; "Top Joggers in Top Jobs," *Newsweek*, July 8, 1968, 60–62; Higdon, "Jogging Is an In Sport," 36–52; Ronald H. Berg, "How Much Jogging Is Good for Your Heart?" *Look*, May 14, 1968, 87–93.

9. "Jogging for Heart and Health—It's Catching On," *U.S. News & World Report*, December 25, 1967, 49; William Zinsser, "The Pious Pad-Pad-Pad of Jogging," *Life*, March 22, 1968, 12; Bill Dellinger, Blaine Newnham, and Warren Morgan, *The Running Experience* (Chicago: Contemporary Books, 1978), viii.

10. Kenneth Cooper, *Aerobics* (New York: M. Evans, 1968).

11. "The Art of Aerobics," *Time*, March 8, 1971, 60.

12. "Udall on the Jog, Opens Jog Trail," *New York Times*, November 8, 1967, 41.

13. "Jogging for Heart and Health," 49.

14. Murray Schumach, "Jogging Picks up Its Pace Here as 20 Tracks Open on Ideal Day," *New York Times*, April 21, 1968, 66.

15. Cooper, *Aerobics*, 1.

16. William Proxmire, *You Can Do It! Senator Proxmire's Exercise, Diet and Relaxation Plan* (New York: Simon & Schuster, 1973), 80.

17. Higdon, "Jogging Is an In Sport," 36–52.

18. Zinsser, "The Pious Pad-Pad-Pad of Jogging," 12.

19. "Don't Just Sit There: Walk, Jog, Run," *Time*, February 23, 1968, 45.

20. Landau, "What Do People Call You?" 28–31.

21. Jean Guarino, "Joggers Need Some Traffic Rules," *Chicago Tribune*, August 22, 1981, S6.

22. Victor F. Zonana, "Joggers and Drivers Have More Run-ins in Streets and Courts," *Wall Street Journal*, March 22, 1978, 1, 25.

23. "Agility Counts, Too," 118–119.

24. Joe Henderson, "Running Commentary," *Runner's World*, March 1976, 12–13.

25. Joe Henderson, "Running Commentary," *Runner's World*, May 1977, 16.

26. "Jogger Regulations Rejected in Jersey," *New York Times*, June 22, 1979, B2.

27. Arthur J. Mollen, "Jay Jogging," *Runner's World*, June 1977, 123; Gary Tuttle, "Running the Light," *Runner's World*, August 1977: 11.

28. Robert Fuston Hall, "Beside the Sidewalks," *Runner's World*, March 1979, 14; Amby Burfoot, "Ambling Along," *Runner's World*, November 1979, 34; Henderson,

"Running Commentary," May 1977, 16; Lisa Gubernick, "Runners Arrested for Jaywalking," *Runner*, June 1979, 11.

29. Richard Hanner, "The Plot against Running," *Runner's World*, April 1978, 52–55. See also Joe Henderson, "Running Commentary," *Runner's World*, April 1978, 20, 23; "A License to Run?" *Running Times*, April 1978, 7.

30. Zonana, "Joggers and Drivers Have More Run-ins," 1, 25.

31. "Under the Wire: Off Limits in Annapolis," *Runner's World*, May 1979, 9.

32. "City Puts Shirt on Their Backs," *Chicago Tribune*, February 11, 1981, 3; "Topless Ban Nearing, Maybe Only on Paper," *New York Times*, February 24, 1981, A14.

33. Karlyn Barker, "Jogger's Paradise Ends," *Washington Post*, April 11, 1979, C1.

34. On violence toward runners, see, for example, Zonana, "Joggers and Drivers Have More Run-ins," 1, 25; Truman R. Clark, "Thugs, Hostile Drivers Have Joggers on the Run," *Los Angeles Times*, June 29, 1978, A19; Robert Anderson, "Origin of Modern Jogger," *Chicago Tribune*, December 8, 1981, A19; Wes Alderson, "Poetic Justice," *Runner's World*, January 1976, 11. One survey found that 75 percent of runners had been the object of hostile remarks from people in passing cars, 63 percent reported having cars intentionally swerve toward them (buzzing), and 33 percent had had objects thrown at them, including cans, bottles, rocks, and firecrackers. "The Runner Census: Part 2: Experiences with Cars," *Running Times*, September 1978, 21–24.

35. Zonana, "Joggers and Drivers Have More Run-ins," 1, 25.

36. Ibid.

37. Ibid.

38. Robert Lipsyte, "Getting into Shape," *New York Times*, June 22, 1968, 37.

39. Clark, "Thugs, Hostile Drivers Have Joggers on the Run," A19.

40. Aristides, "Running and Other Vices," *American Scholar* 48, 2 (1979): 155–163.

41. Higdon, "Proud to Be a Jogger," 29–31.

42. Susan Foster, "Hot Dog Running," *Runner's World*, January 1979, 18.

43. David Zinman, "Bringing out the Runner in Everyone," *Runner's World*, April 1977, 38.

44. James M. Shea, introduction to *Jogging*, by Bowerman and Harris, 3.

45. Richard Bohannon, introduction to *Aerobics*, by Cooper, x.

46. Gerald Besson, "Inner Workings of the Female Runner," *Runner's World*, January 1979, 62–67.

47. Richard Benyo, *Return to Running* (Mt. View, Calif.: World Publications, 1978).

48. B. McClellan, "World's Toughest Runners: Meet the Tarahumara Indians," *Runner's World*, October 1979, 82–84; James F. Fixx, *The Complete Book of Running*

(New York: Random House, 1977). Christopher McDougall's 2009 book is evidence of the continued fascination with this group. Christopher McDougall, *Born to Run: A Hidden Tribe, Superathletes and the Greatest Race the World Has Never Seen* (New York: Knopf, 2009).

49. "Man vs. Machine," *Runner's World*, April 1978, back cover.

50. According to Andrew Kirk, "machines" were not only literal symbols of mobility but also, for the counterculture, metaphors for "a seemingly out-of-control capitalist system." Andrew G. Kirk, *Counterculture Green: The Whole Earth Catalog and American Environmentalism* (Lawrence: University Press of Kansas, 2007), 27.

51. David Corbin, "The Last Laugh," *Runner's World*, February 1974, 8–9.

52. "A Bit of Independence," *Runner's World*, August 1979, back cover.

53. See, for example, Pat Tarnawsky, "Pounding Ground on Earth Day," *Runner's World*, May 1971, 30–31; Edward Ayres, "Aerobic Disposal: Getting out the Mental Garbage," *Running Times*, March 1977, 17–18.

54. Warren Belasco, *Appetite for Change: How the Counterculture Took on the Food Industry* (Ithaca, N.Y.: Cornell University Press, 1989), 30–31.

55. *Running Times*, April 1979, 13.

56. Corbin, "The Last Laugh," 8–9.

57. Barry Commoner, *The Closing Circle: Nature, Man and Technology* (New York: Knopf, 1972); E. F. Schumacher, *Small Is Beautiful: Economics as if People Mattered* (1973; reprint, New York: Harper & Row, 1989); Paul Ehrlich, *The End of Affluence* (New York: Ballantine, 1974); Frances Moore Lappé, *Diet for a Small Planet* (New York: Ballantine, 1975). These works are cited as evidence of cultural change in Paul Boyer, *Promises to Keep: The United States since World War II* (Lexington, Mass.: D. C. Heath, 1995), 380.

58. Daniel Sack, *Whitebread Protestants: Food and Religion in American Culture* (New York: St. Martin's Press, 2000); Belasco, *Appetite for Change*.

59. Jeff Coven, "Where Have All the Marchers Gone?" *Running Times*, June 1978, 18–19.

60. Christopher Lasch, *The Culture of Narcissism: American Life in an Age of Diminishing Expectations* (New York: Norton, 1978).

61. Peter G. Filene, *Into the Arms of Others: A Cultural History of the Right-to-Die in America* (Chicago: Ivan R. Dee, 1998), 65–66.

62. Carll Tucker, "Fear of Dearth," *Saturday Review*, October 27, 1979, 60.

63. Paul J. Kiell and Joseph S. Frelinghuysen, *Keep Your Heart Running: A Graduated, Total Health and Fitness Program for People of All Ages* (New York: Winchester Press, 1976), 35.

64. Curtis Mitchell, *The Joy of Jogging* (New York: Rutledge Books, 1968), 11.

65. Caroline Seebohm, "Running—The New High," *House and Garden*, July 1977, 98, 117.

66. "There Is No Finish Line," *Runner's World*, July 1978, back cover.

67. Letter from Mike Wigal, *Running Times*, January 1979, 6.

68. Letter from Caleb Murdock, *Running Times*, January 1979, 6.

69. "Off the Walt," *Jogger*, December 1979, 3. The existence of the phenomenon continues to be debated; see, for example, Lenny Bernstein, "Runner's High: A Myth Dashed?" *Washington Post*, June 16, 2011, LL13.

70. Leo Diporta, *Zen Running* (New York: Everest House, 1977); Fred Rohé, *The Zen of Running* (New York: Random House, 1974); Joel Henning, *Holistic Running: Beyond the Threshold of Fitness* (New York: Atheneum, 1978); Mike Spino, *Beyond Jogging: The Innerspaces of Running* (Millbrae, Calif.: Celestial Arts, 1976).

71. Higdon, "Is Running a Religious Experience?" 75–79; Ed Jackson, "The Religion Called Running," *Jogger*, December 1979–January 1980, 25; Dick Lawless, "From the Sublime to the Ridiculous," *Footnotes*, Winter 1978, 16; Vic Gold, "The Agnostic Runner," *National Review*, December 8, 1978, 1554–1555; Dick Lawless, "George Sheehan and the Religion of Running," *Footnotes*, Fall 1978, 18.

72. Henning, *Holistic Running*, 1.

73. Haydn Gilmore, *Jog for Your Life* (Grand Rapids, Mich.: Pyranee Books, 1974); Ted Frederick, *Running the Race: The Spiritual Benefits of Running* (Grand Rapids, Mich.: Baker Book House, 1979).

74. Frederick, *Running the Race*, 107.

75. *See How She Runs*, directed by Richard T. Heffron for CBS, aired February 1, 1978. The following year, Michael Douglas appeared in the movie *Running* (directed by Steven Hilliard Stern, Universal Pictures, 1979), which has a similar message that running can lead to a better personal life.

76. Jim Gregoire, "Running out the Door to Sanity," *Runner's World*, July 1978, 41.

77. Kenneth Fox, "On the Run from Alcohol and Other Demons," *Runner's World*, October 1975.

78. Paul de Bruhl, "Escaping the Mind's Prison," *Runner's World*, October 1973, 12–13; Eddie Jenkins, "No Real Prison," *Runner's World*, August 1978, 22; Louie Mendoza, "Running behind Bars," *Footnotes*, Winter 1978, 18; Richard Long, "Running behind Bars: The Best Way to Survive Prison Is to Run through It," *Runner's World*, May 1979, 52–56.

79. *The Jericho Mile*, directed by Michael Mann, ABC Circle Films, aired March 18, 1979.

80. When Dr. Raymond Fowler announced in the *Monitor*, the American Psychological Association's newsletter, that he was organizing an association of

therapists who used running as a mode of treatment, he garnered more than 200 responses. See "Psyched Out," *Runner*, October 1978, 8.

81. William Glasser, *Positive Addiction* (New York: Harper & Row, 1976), 1.

82. Thaddeus Kostrubala, *The Joy of Running* (Philadelphia: J. B. Lippincott, 1976).

83. Valerie Andrews, *The Psychic Power of Running* (New York: Ballantine, 1978), 65.

84. Frank Deford, "Viewpoint," *Sports Illustrated*, June 5, 1978, 10–11.

85. Vic Ziegel and Lewis Grossburger, *The Non-Runner's Book* (New York: Macmillan, 1978).

86. Colman McCarthy, "Biting the Backlash," *Runner*, October 1978, 104.

87. James F. Fixx, "What Running Can't Do for You," *Newsweek*, December 18, 1978, 21.

88. John Kifner, "Thump . . . Thump . . . Gasp . . . Sound of Joggers Increases in the Land," *New York Times*, June 10, 1975, 24.

89. "The Jogging Shoe Race Heats Up," *Business Week*, April 9, 1979, 124–125.

90. Unattributed cartoon, *Jogger*, November 1979, 26.

91. Rosemary Lopez, "Today's Joggers Keep Pace with Style," *New York Times*, September 25, 1977, 416; Ray Dobson, "Fashion on the Run," *New York Times*, July 3, 1977, 256; Nicholas King, "The Jog-Alongs," *National Review*, August 17, 1979, 1034.

92. "The Jogging Shoe Race Heats Up," 124–125.

93. Bowerman and Harris, *Jogging*, 9, 43, 56.

94. Peter Stoler, "Jotters' World," *Time*, August 20, 1979, 72–73.

95. Bob Anderson, "From the Editor," *Runner's World*, December 1979, 7.

96. Len Wallach, *The Human Race: Bay to Breakers Largest Run for Fun in the World* (San Francisco: California Living, 1978), 164, 190.

97. Neil Amdur, "Running Boom: Too Much Too Soon," *New York Times*, April 17, 1978, C1, 8.

98. Quoted in "They're on to Us," *Running Times*, August 1979, 8.

99. Edward Ayres, "Selling Your Body for $3.50," *Running Times*, August 1978, 14–16.

100. R. L. Bohannon, "The Great Beer Bust," *Jogger*, February 1979, 4; "Beer and Running: A Natural Connection," *Running Review*, May 1978, 44; "Run Like a Natural," *Running Review*, May 1978, 45.

101. Dave Collins, "Letters to the Editor," *Running Times*, January 1979, 6.

102. Paul J. Kiell, "Open Letter to Jim Fixx," *Running Times*, September 1979, 6.

103. Carol Krucoff, "Running Fixxations," *Washington Post*, May 8, 1980, C5.

104. Joe Henderson, "Running Commentary," *Runner's World*, August 1977, 25.

105. Janet Heinonen, "Women's Wear for Running," *Runner's World*, May 1974, 28–29.

106. Bob Anderson, "From the Publisher," *Runner's World*, January 1977, 5.

107. George Sheehan, "Medical Advice," *Runner's World*, May 1977, 28.

108. Pamela Cooper, *The American Marathon* (Syracuse, N.Y.: Syracuse University Press, 1998), 139–156.

109. Ibid., 145.

110. Laverne Paradise, "Power-Feminist-Winter Olympics and Weights," *Jogger*, January–February 1976, 3, 9.

111. Susan Cheever Cowley, "Women on the Run," *Newsweek*, November 14, 1977, 100.

112. See, for example, Pat Tarnawsky, "Women vs. the Myths," *Runner's World*, March 1971, 16–17.

113. Katherine Heaviside, "Woman on the Move—At Ten Minutes a Mile," *Redbook*, September 1978, 46, 48.

114. Kay Gilman, "Celebrating Joggers," *Vogue*, October 1978, 52.

115. Elaine Pinkerton, "Women's Running," *Runner's World*, April 1979, 46.

116. "Joggers Run," *New Sign*, April 1969, 1–2; "YMCA Joggers Set for 125 Mile Jaunt," *New York Amsterdam News*, December 14, 1968; "Motorcade and Openhouse Kicks off Harlem 'Y' Campaign," *New Sign*, October 1969, 1–2.

117. Jane Leavy and Susan Okie, "The Runner: Phenomenon of the 70s," *Washington Post*, September 30, 1979, D1, 15.

118. Cited in Cooper, *The American Marathon*, 101.

119. Robert Samuels, "A Hoodie Owner's Decision Calculus," *Washington Post*, April 6, 2012, B2; Cooper, *The American Marathon*, 101.

120. Hugh Coffman, "A Funny Thing Happened on the Way around the Track," *Running Times*, December 1977, 11; "Black Distance Runners: Minority within a Minority," *Runner's World*, January 1976, 37.

121. Don Sabo and Sue Curry Jansen, "Seen But Not Heard: Images of Black Men in Sports Media," in *Sex, Violence and Power in Sports*, ed. Michael A. Messner and Donald F. Sabo (Freedom, Calif.: Crossing Press, 1994), 151–152; David L. Andrews, "Excavating Michael Jordan's Blackness," in *Reading Sport: Critical Essays on Power and Representation*, ed. Susan Birrell and Mary G. McDonald (Boston: Northeastern University Press, 2000), 166–205; Katherine M. Jamieson, "Reading Nancy Lopez," ibid., 144–165.

122. Cooper, *The American Marathon*, 101–102.

123. Leavy and Okie, "The Runner: Phenomenon of the 70s," D1, 15.

124. Carlyle C. Douglas, "Diogenes Put down Your Lantern," *Ebony*, April 1970, 70–79; Carlyle C. Douglas, "Mine Is the Simplest Diet in the World," *Ebony*, February 1977, 64–70; "Jogging Not Harmful to Black Women; It's Dangerous to White Women," *Jet*, July 26, 1979, 54; "Braless Joggers Hurt Own Breasts, Others' Autos," *Jet*, November 23, 1978, 18; "Kitt Sizzles on Broadway," *Jet*, August 31, 1978, 22–24; "Jogging: How to Have Fun Keeping Fit," *Jet*, March 29, 1979, 22–23.

125. Surveys of runner demographics have been reported in Dean C. Jones, "Social Runners," *Runner's World*, July 1976, 6; Frances Knowles, "What Drives the Average Runner?" *Runner's World*, February 1976, 74–75; Frances Knowles, "Women Who Run for Themselves," *Runner's World*, July 1976, 54–55; Anderson, "From the Publisher," 5; "NJA Membership Survey Results," *Jogger*, December 1979–January 1980, 26.

126. Joe Henderson, "An Honest Day's Work," *Runner's World*, October 1974, 18–19.

127. C. P. Gilmore, "Taking Exercise to Heart," *New York Times Magazine*, March 27, 1977, 38–44, 81.

128. Muriel R. Gillick, "Health Promotion, Jogging, and the Pursuit of the Moral Life," *Journal of Health Politics, Policy and Law* 9, 3 (1984): 369–387.

129. J. E. Schmidt, "Jogging Can Kill You . . . and That's Not the Half of It," *Playboy*, March 1976, 87, 152–153.

130. Peter J. Steincrohn, *How to Cure Your Joggermania* (Cranbury, N.J.: A. S. Barnes, 1979), 17, 115–206.

131. Robert Gene Fineberg, *Jogging: The Dance of Death* (Port Washington, N.Y.: Ashley Books, 1980).

132. See, for example, Siegfried J. Kra, "Jogging Is Fine, But Rx Is Caution," *New York Times*, March 11, 1979, C18; Lawrence Meyer, "Byron's Death Raises Runner Alarm," *Washington Post*, October 13, 1978, E1; "Is Jogging Really Good for You?" *U.S. News & World Report*, March 19, 1979, 55–56.

133. See, for example, Sydney H. Schanberg, "It's Sitting Still That's Risky," *New York Times*, August 18, 1984, 23.

134. Russell Baker, "Jogging," *New York Times Magazine*, June 18, 1978, 3; W. Fred Graham, "The Anxiety of the Runner: Terminal Helplessness," *Christian Century*, August 29–September 5, 1979, 821–823; "Justifying Inactivity," *National Review*, June 8, 1979, 763. Death was such a popular topic in jogging literature because a number of cultural and technological developments in the 1970s had led to a reconsideration of what constitutes a good death. The publication of Elizabeth Kubler-Ross's *On Death and Dying* (New York: Macmillan, 1969), the expansion of the hospice movement in the United States, the Karen Ann Quinlan court battle,

and the evolution of the concept of "brain death" as a result of technological innovations that could prolong life indefinitely prompted Americans to rethink the notion of dying with dignity.

135. Thomas J. Bassler, "Marathon Running and Immunity to Heart Disease," *Physician and Sports Medicine* 3, 4 (1975): 77–80. See also James Gorman, "A Running Argument," *Sciences* 17, 1 (1977): 10–15.

136. Bayard Webster, "Running Is Debated as Benefit to Heart," *New York Times*, October 20, 1976, 20.

137. Richard A. Knox, "Even Heart Attack Victims Run in the Boston Marathon," *Washington Post*, April 18, 1974, D6.

138. Joe Henderson, "New Fear in Our Hearts," *Runner's World*, January 1974, 26–28.

139. Gillick, "Health Promotion, Jogging, and the Pursuit of the Moral Life," 369–387.

140. "Is Jogging Really Good for You?" 55–56. Friedman's research was published in Meyer Friedman and Ray H. Rosenman, "Instantaneous and Sudden Death," *Journal of the American Medical Association* 22, 11 (1973): 1319–1328.

141. Paul Starr, *The Social Transformation of American Medicine* (New York: Basic Books, 1982), 389–392; James Whorton, *Nature Cures: The History of Alternative Medicine in America* (Oxford: Oxford University Press, 2002), 245–249.

142. Boston Women's Health Collective, *Our Bodies, Ourselves* (New York: Simon & Schuster, 1973); Whorton, *Nature Cures*, 256–265, 283–288.

143. Higdon, "Proud to Be a Jogger," 30; George Sheehan, "How to Handle Your Enemy, the Doctor," *Footnotes*, Spring 1976, 2; George Sheehan, *Dr. Sheehan on Running* (New York: Bantam, 1978); Darcy C. Plymire, "Running, Heart Disease, and the Ironic Death of Jim Fixx," *Research Quarterly for Exercise and Sport* 73, 1 (2002): 38–46.

144. U.S. Department of Health, Education, and Welfare, *Healthy People: The Surgeon General's Report on Health Promotion and Disease Prevention* (Washington, D.C.: U.S. Government Printing Office, 1979), v, viii.

145. R. L. Bohannon, "Letter to the Editor," *Time*, October 6, 1978, 4–6.

146. Bill Palmer, "National Jogging Day: A Celebration to Fit the Times," *Jogger*, October 1979, 15.

147. "Udall on the Jog, Opens Jog Trail," 41.

148. "Senator Dick Lugar Looks at the Jogging Movement," *Jogger*, June 1978, 7.

149. "You May Be in Prime Condition," *Runner's World*, May 1979, 43.

150. Edward Ayres, "The Authoritarian Runner," *Running Times*, May 1978, 14–16.

CHAPTER 5. TEMPLES OF THE BODY

1. Colman McCarthy, "Running into Trouble," *Washington Post*, September 18, 1979, A19.

2. See, for example, B. Drummond Ayres, "Carter, Exhausted and Pale, Drops out of 6-Mile Race," *New York Times*, September 17, 1979, 1, 40; Jim Mann, "Tiring Carter Forced to Quit 6.2-Mile Race at Midpoint," *Los Angeles Times*, September 16, 1979, 1, 16; Colman McCarthy, "An Uphill Fight for Carter," *Runner*, November 1979, 22–23; Edward Ayres, "Try It Again, Jimmy!" *Running Times*, December 1979, 25.

3. "Was the Post Running On? [letters to the editor]," *Washington Post*, September 20, 1979, A20; Colman McCarthy, "Carter Collapse in Road Race: Symbol of Much, Much More," *Los Angeles Times*, September 20, 1979, E7; Lou Levy, "Jogging Allegory," *Los Angeles Times*, October 1, 1979, C6; Ayres, "Try It Again, Jimmy!" 25.

4. McCarthy, "An Uphill Fight for Carter," 22–23.

5. Mark Shields, "Memo to Jimmy Carter," *Washington Post*, September 5, 1980, A11. Carter continued to exercise, hoping to project an image of both toughness and youth. On vacation in Plains, Georgia, he played tennis and softball and went jogging in 100-degree heat. Locals in Plains favorably compared Carter's physical condition to Reagan's. Brother Billy Carter unwittingly admitted to the press, "He's really showing off now." Eleanor Randolph, "Carter Makes a Point of Exercise in Georgia Heat," *Los Angeles Times*, July 8, 1980, C1, 9.

6. Ronald Reagan, "How to Stay Fit," *Parade*, December 4, 1983, 4–6. See also "So, Move over, Jane Fonda," *Time*, December 12, 1983, 27.

7. This is not to say that exercise denouncers didn't exist. See, for example, Henry A. Solomon, *The Exercise Myth* (San Diego: Harcourt, Brace, Jovanovich, 1984).

8. Charles Leerhsen, "The New Flex Appeal," *Newsweek*, May 6, 1985, 82–83.

9. This chapter uses the terms *gym*, *health club*, and *fitness center* interchangeably. In the 1980s, these terms were virtually indistinguishable, with the exception that only *gym* could designate a venue for competitive or serious bodybuilding or weight lifting. These facilities usually offered few, if any, group fitness classes and little cardiovascular training equipment.

10. David Brand, "A Nation of Health Worrywarts?" *Time*, July 25, 1988, 66.

11. Nicolaus Mills, ed., *Culture in an Age of Money: The Legacy of the 1980s in America* (Chicago: Ivan R. Dee, 1990), 23.

12. John S. Lang, "America's Fitness Binge," *U.S. News & World Report*, May 3, 1982, 58–61.

13. Harvey Green, *Fit for America: Health, Fitness, Sport and American Society* (Baltimore: Johns Hopkins University Press, 1988), 182.

14. Shelly McKenzie, "Athletic Clubs," in *Sports in America from Colonial Times to the Twenty-First Century: An Encyclopedia*, ed. Steven A. Riess (Armonk, N.Y.: Sharpe Online Reference, 2011). While athletic clubs flourished, companion establishments that provided facilities for the working class also proliferated. The YMCA, YWCA, YMHA, and YWHA, along with institutional churches and settlement houses, provided designated spaces for physical conditioning, albeit in more modest settings.

15. "Fat," *Newsweek*, July 27, 1959, 76–77.

16. "The Long Odds," *Tightrope*, directed by Oscar Rudolph, aired February 16, 1960; "Bob the Body Builder," *The Bob Cummings Show*, directed by Bob Cummings, aired November 12, 1957; "Jack Goes to the Gym," *The Jack Benny Show*, aired February 5, 1961; "Beautiful Dreamer," *The Green Hornet*, directed by Allen Reisner, aired July 7 (part 1) and 14 (part 2), 1967.

17. A few health clubs along the lines of turn-of-the-century athletic clubs continued to exist and provided cultural models for middle-class clubs to emulate. See, for example, "Los Angeles Limbers Up," *Sports Illustrated*, January 2, 1956, 42–43; "Construction Under Way for Health Club Building," *Los Angeles Times*, April 18, 1954, E10.

18. Thomas Buckley, "State Is Studying Vic Tanny Losses," *New York Times*, December 11, 1963, 1; Peter Bunzel, "Health Kick's High Priest," *Life*, September 29, 1958, 71–75; "Fat," 76–77.

19. Bunzel, "Health Kick's High Priest," 71–75.

20. "Fat," 76–77.

21. "Chain Site Hunt Is Intricate Job," *New York Times*, May 27, 1958, 53.

22. "The Tanny Tumble," *Newsweek*, December 23, 1963, 60; Stanley Frank, "Illusions of Reducing," *Saturday Evening Post*, January 20, 1962, 28–31.

23. Josh Buck, "The Evolution of Health Clubs," *Club Industry*, December 1999, 16–18; Frank, "Illusions of Reducing," 28–31.

24. "Desk Fatigue? Renew Your Health and Vigor," *Los Angeles Times*, August 12, 1957, C3; "I Gained 55 Pounds of Muscle in 6 Months," *Los Angeles Times*, February 24, 1958, C4; "Be the Man of Her Ideals," *Los Angeles Times*, August 9, 1957, C5. Delmonteque was a bodybuilder who had posed for physique magazines earlier in his career. See Valentine Hooven, *Beefcake: The Muscle Magazines of America, 1950–1970* (Berlin: Taschen Verlag, 1996), 66, 122.

25. For images of the chronological development of muscular stars in Hollywood, see David L. Chapman and Brett Josef Grubisic, *American Hunks: The Muscular Male Body in American Culture* (Vancouver: Arsenal Pulp Press, 2009); Hooven, *Beefcake*.

26. Frank, "Illusions of Reducing," 28–31.

27. Dena Kaye, "Spring Shape-up Guide," *New York Times Magazine*, March 27, 1977, 215; Angela Taylor, "For Those Whose Goals Are Firm Muscles and a Svelte Body," *New York Times*, September 16, 1974, 49.

28. Winzola McLendon, "One Big Money Maker Prefers Losses to Gains for Customers," *Washington Post*, August 17, 1958, C8.

29. Ibid.

30. Agnes McCarty, "Those Salons of Reducing Offer Expanding Careers," *New York Times*, April 5, 1956, 32; Ruth Wagner, "Figure Problems Add up to Her Job," *Washington Post*, July 1, 1956, F9.

31. For more on the magic couch, see Peter Wyden, *The Overweight Society* (New York: Pocket Books, 1965), 216–218.

32. McCarty, "Those Salons of Reducing Offer Expanding Careers," 32; "Slimming for Slenderella," *Time*, May 4, 1959, time.com, accessed July 27, 2007.

33. Winzola McLendon, "Got a Weighty Problem? Then Take It Lying Down," *Washington Post*, August 22, 1957, C13.

34. Ibid.; McLendon, "One Big Money Maker Prefers Losses to Gains," C8.

35. Harry Gabbett, "Round 9000 Weights Here," *Washington Post*, May 1, 1959, C13.

36. Ruth Wagner, "First Time They Saw Paris," *Washington Post*, March 13, 1959, D7.

37. "From Size 20 to 14 for Keeps: Advertisement for Slenderella," *Washington Post*, January 23, 1952, B6.

38. McLendon, "Got a Weighty Problem?" C13.

39. "The Pink Jungle," *Time*, June 16, 1958, time.com, accessed May 23, 2012.

40. For more on the influence of space travel and automation on midcentury popular culture, see Thomas Hine, *Populuxe* (New York: Knopf, 1986), chaps. 5–8.

41. Even though effortless exercise had been largely discredited by the 1970s, it never completely vanished. As late as 1982, the *Advocate* touted the opening of a "new" kind of gym in Los Angeles that employed electric stimulation for body shaping and weight loss. William Franklin, "Passive Exercise and the New Moderns," *Advocate*, August 19, 1982, 53.

42. The brochure is attached as appendix KK in Harold T. Friermood, "Health Clubs in the YMCA with Respect to Current Status and Development of Operating Standards" (Ed.D. diss., New York University, 1954), 426.

43. Barney Lefferts, "Swanky Sweatshops," *New York Times Magazine*, March 23, 1958, 47–48.

44. Ibid.

45. Taylor, "For Those Whose Goals Are Firm Muscles and a Svelte Body," 49.

46. Margaret Roach, "A Few Good Places to Get in Shape," New York Times, July 10, 1978, C10.

47. See Clarence G. Lasby, Eisenhower's Heart Attack: How Ike Beat Heart Disease and Held On to the Presidency (Lawrence: University Press of Kansas, 1996); Barbara Ehrenreich, The Hearts of Men: American Dreams and the Flight from Commitment (Garden City, N.Y.: Anchor Press, 1983), 66–87.

48. Eugene B. Mozes, Living beyond Your Heart Attack (Englewood Cliffs, N.J.: Prentice-Hall, 1959), 83.

49. "Keeping Fit in the Company Gym," Fortune, October 1975, 139–143.

50. David Rees Brown, "Sweating It Out: Desk-Bound Executives Decide that Exercise Is Worth the Effort," Wall Street Journal, May 2, 1968, 1; Eric Morganthaler, "In the Pink: Stereotype of Unfit Overweight Executive Turns Out to Be Wrong," Wall Street Journal, May 21, 1971, 1; "Keeping Fit in the Company Gym," 139–143; Alexandra Penney, "Shaping Up the Corporate Image," New York Times Magazine, October 7, 1979, 21; Elaine Budd, "Physical Fitness as a Fringe Benefit," New York Times, April 1, 1979, WC14; Robert Enstad, "Keeping Fit: It Gives an On-the-Job Lift," Chicago Tribune, August 5, 1979, P14.

51. Penney, "Shaping Up the Corporate Image," 21–22; Sandy Rovner, "Health Talk: Corporate Fitness," Washington Post, August 31, 1979, C5.

52. Carol Oppenheim, "Physical Conditioning Fits Right In with Business Ideas," Chicago Tribune, September 7, 1978, A7.

53. Solomon, The Exercise Myth, 4; Rovner, "Health Talk: Corporate Fitness," C5.

54. Howard Reich, "Staying in Shape, out of Town," Chicago Tribune, April 18, 1979, F1; Stephen Birnbaum, "Where to Go for a Hotel—Plus Exercise," Chicago Tribune, October 25, 1981, K15.

55. "How to Stop from Going to Pot," Time, May 30, 1969, 80.

56. Leslie Bennetts, "American Capitalism Sees the Profit in Physical Fitness," New York Times, June 12, 1978, B14.

57. Brown, "Sweating It Out," 1; Morganthaler, "In the Pink," 1; John Getze, "Executives Sweat to Save Their Companies Money," Los Angeles Times, October 5, 1975, G1, 5; John Cavanaugh, "On the Corporate Treadmill," New York Times, March 11, 1979, CN1; Milt Freudenheim, "Assessing the Corporate Fitness Craze," New York Times, March 18, 1990, F1, 6.

58. "Top Joggers in Top Jobs," Newsweek, July 8, 1968, 60–62.

59. "Experts at Rat Race Get Chance to Show Stuff on a Real Track," Wall Street Journal, September 22, 1972, 16.

60. Bennetts, "American Capitalism Sees the Profit in Physical Fitness," B14.

61. Cited in Marc Stern, "The Fitness Movement and the Fitness Center Industry, 1960–2000" (paper presented at the BHC annual meeting, 2008, Business and Economic History On-line).

62. "Fat People's Fight against Job Bias," U.S. News & World Report, December 5, 1977, 80.

63. Laurie Baum, "Extra Pounds Can Weigh Down Your Career," Business Week, August 3, 1987, 96.

64. "Fat People's Fight against Job Bias," 78–80.

65. Jane E. Brody, "Personal Health," New York Times, November 27, 1985, C7; Freudenheim, "Assessing the Corporate Fitness Craze," F1.

66. Weight lifting and bodybuilding, at an elite level, designate different activities. The goal of weight lifting is to lift progressively heavier weights in different poses. The focus of bodybuilding is the development of a symmetrical, proportioned musculature. Unlike weight lifting, which is a recognized Olympic sport, detractors of bodybuilding claim that it is not a sport. Many original sources use these two terms indiscriminately. Both these activities influenced amateur exercisers working out in gyms in the 1970s and 1980s.

67. Charles Gaines and George Butler, Pumping Iron: The Art and Sport of Bodybuilding (New York: Simon & Schuster, 1974); Pumping Iron, directed by George Butler and Robert Fore, White Mountain Films, 1977.

68. John Cassidy, "Still Pumped Up," New Yorker, November 25, 2002, new yorker.com, accessed September 2, 2007.

69. Michaelangelo Signorile, Life Outside: The Signorile Report on Gay Men: Sex, Drugs, Muscles, and the Passages of Life (New York: HarperCollins, 1997), 53.

70. Martin P. Levine, Gay Macho: The Life and Death of the Homosexual Clone (New York: New York University Press, 1998), 59–60.

71. Ibid., 61, 65.

72. Gil Troy, Morning in America: How Ronald Reagan Invented the 1980s (Princeton, N.J.: Princeton University Press, 2005), 218–220; Lynne Luciano, Looking Good: Male Body Image in America (New York: Hill & Wang, 2001), 154.

73. Dominique Padurano, "Making American Men: Charles Atlas and the Business of Bodies, 1892–1945" (Ph.D. diss., Rutgers University, 2007), 211–220.

74. Quoted in Kenneth Dutton, The Perfectible Body: The Western Idea of Physical Development (London: Cassell, 1995), 145.

75. Gaines and Butler, Pumping Iron, 90, 92.

76. Lynn Darling, "How Much Bigger Can Arnold Schwarzenegger Get?" Esquire, March 1985, 128–132.

77. Levine, Gay Macho, 71–72.

78. Signorile, *Life Outside*, xix, 60.

79. Lenny Giteck, "The Gay Pursuit of Muscle," *Advocate*, June 11, 1981, 27.

80. Gaines and Butler, *Pumping Iron*, 60, 72–74.

81. Ibid., 76–77. Samuel Fussell's chronicle of the Southern California bodybuilding scene in the 1980s similarly describes rampant steroid use. Samuel Fussell, *Muscle: Confessions of an Unlikely Bodybuilder* (New York: Poseidon Press, 1991), 117–123. On the general unhealthiness of competitive bodybuilding, see also Luciano, *Looking Good*, 151–152.

82. Alexandra Penney, "Showing Some New Muscle," *New York Times Magazine*, June 15, 1980, 15.

83. My thanks to Francisco Soto for drawing my attention to this important development. See also "Machines for Pumping Iron," *New York Times*, July 25, 1982, F7; "The Case for Nautilus: 'Full Range' Exercise," *New York Times*, July 10, 1978, C10.

84. "The Case for Nautilus," C10.

85. Andrew Sullivan, "Muscleheads," *New Republic*, September 15–22, 1986, 24.

86. Steven Findlay, "Smart Ways to Shape Up," *U.S. News & World Report*, July 18, 1988, 46–49.

87. Anastasia Toufexis, "The Shape of the Nation," *Time*, October 7, 1985, 60–61.

88. Raquel Welch, *Raquel: The Raquel Welch Total Beauty and Fitness Program* (New York: Holt, Rinehart & Winston, 1984); John Travolta, *Staying Fit! His Complete Program for Reshaping Your Body through Weight Resistance Training and Modern Dance Techniques* (New York: Simon & Schuster, 1984); Linda Evans, *Linda Evans' Beauty and Exercise Book* (New York: Simon & Schuster, 1983); Victoria Principal, *The Body Principal* (New York: Simon & Schuster, 1983); Jayne Kennedy, *Love Your Body and More: Jayne Kennedy's Advanced Exercise Program* (Nashville: Compleat Records, 1982); Marie Osmond, *Marie Osmond's Exercises for Mothers-to-Be* (New York: New American Library, 1985); Jane Fonda, *Jane Fonda's Workout Book* (New York: Simon & Schuster, 1981).

89. David Ferrell, "Joe Weider's Iron Grip on an Empire," *Los Angeles Times*, March 2, 1989, 1, 24.

90. Jack McCallum, "Everybody's Doin' It," *Sports Illustrated*, December 3, 1984, 72–86.

91. On the militaristic strain in Ronald Reagan's presidency, see Michael Schaller, *Reckoning with Reagan: America and Its President in the 1980s* (New York: Oxford University Press, 1992), 119–147.

92. Dutton, *The Perfectible Body*, 212–213.

93. Shields, "Memo to Jimmy Carter," A11.

94. Susan Jeffords, *Hard Bodies: Hollywood Masculinity in the Reagan Era* (New Brunswick, N.J.: Rutgers University Press, 1994), 24.

95. *First Blood*, directed by Ted Kotcheff, Orion Pictures, 1982; *Rambo: First Blood Part II*, directed by George Cosmatos, Tristar Pictures, 1985; *Rambo III*, directed by Peter MacDonald, Artisan Entertainment, 1988. Sylvester Stallone's physical appearance as Rambo suggested his previous role as Rocky Balboa in *Rocky* (1976) and *Rocky II* (1979). Both those films, set in the world of boxing, were evidence of the physical turn taken by popular culture at the end of the 1970s. Unlike *First Blood*, however, they exhibited a particularly working-class sensibility, in line with the decade's "blue-collar revival." For example, for Tony Manero, the dance champion of *Saturday Night Fever* (1977), physical culture represented an opportunity to demonstrate worthiness through competition, unlike middle-class fitness pursuits, which were typically more inner directed. Jefferson Cowie, "'Vigorously Left, Right and Center': The Crosscurrents of Working-Class America in the 1970s," in *America in the 70s*, ed. Beth Bailey and David Farber (Lawrence: University Press of Kansas, 2004), 76.

96. Jeffords, *Hard Bodies*, 28.

97. Hal Higdon, "Training," *Runner*, August 1982, 52–53.

98. Chris Cobbs, "You Might Call It Survival of the Fittest," *Los Angeles Times*, December 3, 1980, B1; "History of Ironman," www.ironmanworldchampionship .com, accessed July 2, 2012.

99. For more on the new intensity, see, for example, Alexandra Penney, "Tough Is Good for You," *New York Times Magazine*, August 14, 1977, 54; Michael Walsh, "Make Way for the New Spartans," *Time*, September 19, 1983, 90–92; "Classes at Seven Top Studios," *New York Times*, May 23, 1984, C10.

100. Walsh, "Make Way for the New Spartans."

101. Wanda Urbanska, *The Singular Generation* (Garden City, N.Y.: Doubleday, 1986), 100.

102. Ray Oldenburg, *The Great Good Place* (New York: Paragon House, 1989).

103. A follow-up book that described new kinds of third places did include gyms. See James Smith, Charles Gourgott, and Patrick Devine, "The Great Good Gym," in *Celebrating the Third Place*, ed. Ray Oldenburg (New York: Marlowe, 2001), 130–140.

104. Findlay, "Smart Ways to Shape Up," 46–49.

105. Martin Hochbaum, "Requiem for Yesterday's Gym," *New York Times*, October 27, 1984, 27.

106. See, for example, John Dietrich and Susan Waggoner, *The Complete Health Club Handbook* (New York: Simon & Schuster, 1983); Robert Lindsey, "Health Clubs

Thrive as Meeting Places for Young Single People," *New York Times*, December 4, 1981, A18; Richard Phillips, "A Consumer's Guide to Health Clubs," *Chicago Tribune*, September 10, 1982, 1–2.

107. See, for example, Rudy Maxa, "A Guide to Area Health Clubs," *Washington Post*, February 13, 1972, 20, 38; Phillips, "A Consumer's Guide to Health Clubs," 1–2; Roach, "A Few Good Places to Get in Shape," C10; Reba Churchill and Bonnie Churchill, "Exercising's Your Option," *Los Angeles Times*, May 4, 1982, I1. In addition, at least two national guides to health clubs were published: Dietrich and Waggoner, *The Complete Health Club Handbook*; Maury Z. Levy and Jay Shafran, *Gym Psych: The Insider's Guide to Health Clubs* (New York: Fawcett Columbine, 1986).

108. Lindsey, "Health Clubs Thrive as Meeting Places," A18.

109. Ibid.

110. Paul Hendrickson, "Among the Believers at the High-Tech Temple of Sweat," *Washington Post*, February 2, 1982, C1, 2.

111. Lindsey, "Health Clubs Thrive as Meeting Places," A18.

112. Michael Denneny, "Hymn to a Gym," *Poz*, May 1997, poz.com, accessed July 7, 2012.

113. Levine, *Gay Macho*, 39–54.

114. Matt Kalkhoff, "The John Blair Project," *New York Blade*, May 23, 2003, nyblade.com, accessed August 25, 2007. Available at www.mattunleashed.com/nyblade_030523.htm as of July 7, 2012.

115. Jan Carl Park, "Free Weights and Free Enterprise," *New York Native*, January 14–27, 1985, 26.

116. Levine, *Gay Macho*, 50.

117. Denneny, "Hymn to a Gym."

118. Signorile, *Life Outside*, 67.

119. David Tuller, "Some Gay Businesses Suffer, Others Thrive in Era of AIDS," *Newsday*, May 2, 1988, 3; David Tuller, "AIDS Crisis Changing Face of Gay Business," *San Francisco Chronicle*, August 29, 1988, C1.

120. Tuller, "Some Gay Businesses Suffer," 3.

121. Denneny, "Hymn to a Gym"; Michael Shernoff, "Scenes from Chelsea Gym," *LGNY*, December 1, 1996.

122. Shernoff, "Scenes from Chelsea Gym."

123. Ibid.

124. Robert D. Putnam, *Bowling Alone: The Collapse and Revival of American Community* (New York: Simon & Schuster, 2000).

125. "Tannyed & Fit," *Time*, February 10, 1961, 76.

126. Ibid.

127. Buckley, "State Is Studying Vic Tanny Losses," 1, 53.

128. Thomas Buckley, "State Acts to Bar Tanny Debt Suits," New York Times, December 17, 1963, 41.

129. Frank, "Illusions of Reducing," 28–31.

130. Gabbett, "Round 9000 Weights Here," C13; "Tax Liens Filed on Slenderella," Washington Post, April 22, 1959, D6; "Slimming for Slenderella."

131. "Beautiful Dreamer," The Green Hornet.

132. Richard B. Schmitt, "Fiscal Fitness: Efforts to Regulate Health Clubs Fail to End Abuses," Wall Street Journal, April 3, 1987, 1.

133. John Darnton, "U.S. Looking at Service Contracts Here," New York Times, June 3, 1971, 14; Grace Lichtenstein, "Fraud Complaints on Health-Spas Rise," New York Times, December 26, 1972, 1, 16; "F.T.C. Investigating Salons and Schools," New York Times, May 6, 1974, 55; "Deception Is Laid to 11 Health Spas," New York Times, July 17, 1974, 73; Carole Shifrin, "FTC Proposes Curbs on Health Clubs," Washington Post, August 17, 1975, C7; Larry Kramer, "Health Spa Regulation Endorsed," Washington Post, May 2, 1979, D6; Molly Sinclair, "Health Clubs: Exercise Your Rights," Washington Post, February 9, 1983, B2; S. J. Diamond, "Health Club Customers Must Exercise Caution," Los Angeles Times, November 5, 1984, E1; Doug Brown, "Some Health Clubs Fail the Fitness Test," Los Angeles Times, April 19, 1984, D1; Schmitt, "Fiscal Fitness," 1; Stern, "The Fitness Movement and the Fitness Center Industry."

134. Friermood, "Health Clubs in the YMCA," 95–105. Friermood's study was based on membership records as of December 31, 1946.

135. "Negro Quits 'Y' Board," New York Times, November 22, 1959, 75.

136. "Club Loses Racial Suit," New York Times, January 24, 1962, 51.

137. "Jazz Pianist McCann Charges Atlanta YMCA Discriminated," Washington Post, June 16, 1967, A4.

138. "Bally's U.S. Health Is Sued by the U.S. on Racial Bias Charge," Wall Street Journal, February 13, 1989, C11; Rochelle Riley, "Area Spas Agree Not to Discriminate," Washington Post, April 28, 1989, C6; "Six Employees of Spa Allege Discrimination," Washington Post, June 15, 1989, B9; Tracy Thompson, "Suit against Holiday Spa Expands," Washington Post, November 14, 1989, D3; Neil A. Lewis, "Rights Group Sues Gyms over Membership," New York Times, November 14, 1989, A25; Paul M. Barrett, "U.S. Court Orders U.S. Health to End Its Discrimination," Wall Street Journal, April 28, 1989, 1; Paul W. Valentine, "Federal Judge Orders Newspaper Ads in Bias Suit against Holiday Spas," Washington Post, November 10, 1990, B4; "In Settling Lawsuit, Health Club Chain Admits Racial Bias," New York Times, March 2, 1991, 10; "Spa Owner to Pay Blacks over Hiring Bias," Washington Post, January 6, 1992.

139. McCallum, "Everybody's Doin' It," 76.

140. Jeff B. Copeland, "Are Health Clubs Risky?" *Newsweek*, February 17, 1986, 62.

141. Karen S. Peterson, "Exercise at Your Own Risk," *Washington Post*, April 17, 1983, A1.

142. Copeland, "Are Health Clubs Risky?" 62; "Debate Grows on Standards for Certifying Fitness Instructors," *New York Times*, March 3, 1988, B7.

143. Anastasia Toufexis, "Watch the Bouncing Body," *Time*, June 30, 1986, 74. For examples of new kinds of workout regimens, see Amy Singer, "Classic Shape-ups," *New York Times Magazine*, March 2, 1982, 56.

144. Barbara Lloyd, "Step up (and down) to Sharper Workouts," *New York Times*, March 26, 1990, C10.

145. Findlay, "Smart Ways to Shape Up," 46–49.

146. Singer, "Classic Shape-ups," 56.

147. John P. Robinson and Geoffrey Godbey, "Has Fitness Peaked?" *American Demographics*, September 1993, 36–42.

148. Joseph Pereira, "The Exercise Boom Loses Its Strength—Jobs, Families Take Priority," *Wall Street Journal*, January 9, 1989, 1.

149. Toufexis, "The Shape of the Nation," 60–61.

150. Blair Sabol, *The Body of America* (New York: Arbor House, 1986), 220–223.

EPILOGUE: THE FUTURE OF FITNESS

1. Peter J. Steincrohn, *How to Be Lazy, Healthy and Fit* (New York: Funk & Wagnalls, 1968), 75.

2. Both these activities have a long history that predates their current vogue. On the history of yoga in the United States, see Stefanie Symon, *The Subtle Body: The Story of Yoga in America* (New York: Farrar, Straus & Giroux, 2010); Robert Love, *The Great Oom: The Improbable Birth of Yoga in America* (New York: Viking, 2010). For the development of Pilates, see Penelope Latey, "History and Philosophy of Pilates," *Journal of Bodywork and Movement Therapies* 5, 4 (2001): 275–282.

3. Expensive yoga gear is one prominent aspect of the "commodification of yoga." Rob Walker, "Marketing Pose," *New York Times Magazine*, July 26, 2009, 18.

4. Paul Kendall, "Yoga and the Art of Making Money," *Sunday Telegraph*, November 6, 2011, 11.

5. Anna Holmes, "Competitive Yoga? Down Dog," *Washington Post*, March 9, 2012, C1, 4.

6. The extent to which yoga has been appropriated by American practitioners is evident in a recent campaign by the Hindu American Foundation to "Take Back

Yoga." Paul Vitello, "Hindu Group Stirs a Debate over Yoga's Soul," *New York Times,* November 28, 2010, A1.

7. Jennifer Smith Maguire, *Fit for Consumption: Sociology and the Business of Fitness* (London: Routledge, 2008), 193.

8. David Riesman, *The Lonely Crowd: A Study of the Changing American Character* (New Haven, Conn.: Yale University Press, 1950).

9. National Center for Health Statistics, *Health, United States: With Special Feature on Socioeconomic Status and Health* (Hyattsville, Md., 2011), 252–256, www.cdc.gov/nchs/data/hus/hus11.pdf.

10. Ross C. Brownson, Tegan K. Boehmer, and Douglas A. Luke, "Declining Rates of Physical Activity in the United States: What Are the Contributors?" *Annual Review of Public Health* 26 (2005): 421–443.

11. Peter A. Katzmarzyk, "Physical Activity, Sedentary Behavior, and Health: Paradigm Paralysis or Paradigm Shift?" *Diabetes* 59, 11 (2010): 2717–2725; W. J. Brown, A. E. Bauman, and N. Owen, "Stand up, Sit down, Keep Moving: Turning in Circles in Physical Activity Research?" *British Journal of Sports Medicine* 43, 2 (2009): 86–88; James A. Levine, "Non-exercise Activity Thermogenesis (NEAT)," *Nutrition Reviews* 62, 7 (2004): S82–S97; James A. Levine, "NEAT," *Best Practice and Research Clinical Endocrinology and Metabolism* 16, 4 (2002): 679–702; Michael S. Rosenwald, "Desk Jockeys Rising Up, Putting Chairs out of a Job," *Washington Post,* October 17, 2010, A1, 18; James Vlhaos, "Is Sitting a Lethal Activity?" *New York Times Magazine,* April 17, 2011, 39.

12. S. W. Ng and B. M. Popkin, "Time Use and Physical Activity: A Shift away from Movement across the Globe," *Obesity Reviews* (2012), doi:10.1111/j.1467-1789X.2011.00982.x, accessed July 13, 2012.

SELECTED BIBLIOGRAPHY

Abrams, Nathan, and Julie Hughes, eds. *Containing America*. Birmingham, U.K.: Birmingham University Press, 2000.

Adams, Mark. *Mr. America: How Muscular Millionaire Bernarr MacFadden Transformed the Nation through Sex, Salad, and the Ultimate Starvation Diet*. New York: Harper-Collins, 2009.

Adams, Mary Louise. *The Trouble with Normal: Postwar Youth and the Making of Heterosexuality*. Toronto: University of Toronto Press, 1997.

Addison, Heather. *Hollywood and the Rise of Physical Culture*. New York: Taylor & Francis, 2003.

Alvarez, Erick. *Muscle Boys: Gay Gym Culture*. New York: Routledge, 2008.

Andrews, David L. "Excavating Michael Jordan's Blackness." In *Reading Sport: Critical Essays on Power and Representation*, ed. Susan Birrell and Mary G. McDonald, 166–205. Boston: Northeastern University Press, 2000.

Bailey, Beth, and David Farber, eds. *America in the 70s*. Lawrence: University Press of Kansas, 2004.

Banner, Lois. *American Beauty*. Chicago: University of Chicago Press, 1983.

Barsky, Arthur J. *Worried Sick: Our Troubled Quest for Wellness*. Boston: Little, Brown, 1988.

Bederman, Gail. *Manliness and Civilization: A Cultural History of Race and Gender in the United States, 1880–1917*. Chicago: University of Chicago Press, 1995.

Belasco, Warren. *Appetite for Change: How the Counterculture Took On the Food Industry*. Ithaca, N.Y.: Cornell University Press, 1989.

Benzie, Tim. "Judy Garland at the Gym—Gay Magazines and Gay Bodybuilding." *Continuum: Journal of Media & Cultural Studies* 14, 2 (2000): 159–170.

Berrett, Jesse. "Feeding the Organization Man: Diet and Masculinity in Postwar America." *Journal of Social History* 30, 4 (Summer 1997): 805–825.

Berryman, Jack W. "Thomas K. Cureton, Jr.: Pioneer Researcher, Proselytizer, and Proponent for Physical Fitness." *Research Quarterly for Exercise and Sport* 67, 1 (1996): 1–12.

Blumenthal, Sidney. "Reaganism and the Neokitsch Aethestic." In *The Reagan Legacy*, ed. Sidney Blumenthal and Thomas Byrne Edsall, 251–294. New York: Pantheon, 1988.

Bordo, Susan. *The Male Body: A New Look at Men in Public and in Private*. New York: Farrar, Straus & Giroux, 1999.

―――. *Unbearable Weight: Feminism, Western Culture and the Body.* Berkeley: University of California Press, 1993.

Borstelmann, Thomas. *The 1970s: A New Global History from Civil Rights to Economic Inequality.* Princeton, N.J.: Princeton University Press, 2012.

Bowerman, William J., and W. E. Harris. *Jogging: A Physical Fitness Program for All Ages.* New York: Grosset & Dunlap, 1967.

Boyer, Paul. *Promises to Keep: The United States since World War II.* Lexington, Mass.: D. C. Heath, 1995.

Braunstein, Peter, and Michael William Doyle, eds. *Imagine Nation: The American Counterculture of the 1960s and 70s.* New York: Routledge, 2002.

Breines, Wini. *Young, White and Miserable: Growing up Female in the Fifties.* 2nd ed. Chicago: University of Chicago Press, 2001.

Brenner, Leslie. *American Appetite.* New York: Avon Books, 1999.

Broadwater, Jeff. *Eisenhower and the Anti-Communist Crusade.* Chapel Hill: University of North Carolina Press, 1992.

Bronzino, Joseph D., Vincent H. Smith, and Maurice L. Wade. *Medical Technology and Society: An Interdisciplinary Perspective.* Cambridge, Mass.: MIT Press, 1990.

Brumburg, Joan Jacobs. *Fasting Girls: The Development of Anorexia Nervosa.* Cambridge, Mass.: Harvard University Press, 1988.

Budd, Michael Anton. *The Sculpture Machine: Physical Culture and Body Politics in the Age of Empire.* New York: New York University Press, 1997.

Carlson, Rick J. *The End of Medicine.* New York: John Wiley, 1975.

Carroll, Peter N. *It Seemed Like Nothing Happened: The Tragedy and Promise of America in the 1970s.* New York: Holt, Rinehart & Winston, 1982.

Carruthers, Susan L. *Cold War Captives: Imprisonment, Escape and Brainwashing.* Berkeley: University of California Press, 2009.

―――. "'The Manchurian Candidate' and the Cold War Brainwashing Scare." *Historical Journal of Film, Radio and Television* 18, 1 (1998): 75–94.

Cassedy, James H. *Medicine in America: A Short History.* Baltimore: Johns Hopkins University Press, 1991.

Cassidy, Marsha F. *What Women Watched: Daytime Television in the 1950s.* Austin: University of Texas Press, 2005.

Chapman, David L., and Brett Josef Grubisic. *American Hunks: The Muscular Male Body in American Culture.* Vancouver: Arsenal Pulp Press, 2009.

Chauncey, George. "Lots of Friends at the YMCA: Rooming Houses, Cafeterias, and Other Gay Social Centers." In *The Gender and Consumer Culture Reader*, ed. Jennifer Scanlon, 49–69. New York: New York University Press, 2000.

Clecak, Peter. *America's Quest for the Ideal Self: Dissent and Fulfillment in the 60s and 70s.* New York: Oxford University Press, 1983.

Clowse, Barbara Barksdale. *Brainpower for the Cold War: The Sputnik Crisis and National Defense Education Act of 1958.* Westport, Conn.: Greenwood Press, 1981.

Cohan, Steven. *Masked Men: Masculinity and the Movies in the Fifties.* Bloomington: Indiana University Press, 1997.

Cohen, Lizabeth. *A Consumer's Republic: The Politics of Mass Consumption in Postwar America.* New York: Knopf, 2003.

Collins, Robert M. *Transforming America: Politics and Culture in the Reagan Years.* New York: Columbia University Press, 2003.

Commoner, Barry. *The Closing Circle: Nature, Man and Technology.* New York: Knopf, 1972.

Coontz, Stephanie. *The Way We Never Were: American Families and the Nostalgia Trap.* New York: Basic Books, 1992.

Cooper, Cary L., and Philip Dewe. *Stress: A Brief History.* Malden, Mass.: Blackwell, 2004.

Cooper, Pamela. *The American Marathon.* Syracuse, N.Y.: Syracuse University Press, 1998.

———. "The 'Visible Hand' on the Footrace: Fred Lebow and the Marketing of the Marathon." *Journal of Sport History* 19, 3 (Winter 1992): 244–257.

Cooter, Roger, and John Pickstone, eds. *Medicine in the Twentieth Century.* Amsterdam: Harwood Academic Publishers, 2000.

Corber, Robert J. *Homosexuality in Cold War America.* Durham, N.C.: Duke University Press, 1997.

———. *In the Name of National Security: Hitchcock, Homophobia, and the Political Construction of Gender in Postwar America.* Durham, N.C.: Duke University Press, 1993.

Cowan, Ruth Schwartz. *More Work for Mother.* New York: Basic Books, 1985.

Crawford, Robert. "Healthism and the Medicalization of Everyday Life." *International Journal of Health Services* 10, 3 (1980): 365–388.

———. "Individual Responsibility and Health Politics in the 1970s." In *Health Care in America,* ed. Susan Reverby and David Rosner, 247–268. Philadelphia: Temple University Press, 1979.

———. "You Are Dangerous to Your Health." *Social Policy* 8, 1 (January–February 1978): 11–20.

Creadick, Anna G. *Perfectly Average: The Pursuit of Normality in Postwar America.* Amherst: University of Massachusetts Press, 2010.

Crosbie, Philip. *March til They Die.* Westminster, Md.: Newman Press, 1956.

Dawber, Thomas Royle. *The Framingham Study: The Epidemiology of Atherosclerotic Disease.* Cambridge, Mass.: Harvard University Press, 1980.

Deane, Philip. *I Was a Captive in Korea.* New York: Norton, 1953.

de la Pena, Carolyn. *Empty Pleasures: The Story of Artificial Sweeteners from Saccharin to Splenda.* Chapel Hill: University of North Carolina Press, 2010.

Divine, Robert A. *The Sputnik Challenge.* New York: Oxford University Press, 1993.

Doherty, Thomas. *Teenagers and Teenpics: The Juvenilization of American Movies in the 1950s.* 2nd ed. Philadelphia: Temple University Press, 2002.

Douglas, Susan J. *Where the Girls Are: Growing up Female with the Mass Media.* New York: Random House, 1994.

Dutton, Kenneth. *The Perfectible Body: The Western Idea of Physical Development.* London: Cassell, 1995.

Dworkin, Shari L., and Faye Linda Wachs. *Body Panic: Gender, Health and the Selling of Fitness.* New York: New York University Press, 2009.

Edelstein, Andrew J., and Kevin McDonough. *The Seventies: From Hot Pants to Hot Tubs.* New York: Dutton, 1990.

Edgley, Charles, and Dennis Brissett. "Health Nazis and the Cult of the Perfect Body: Some Polemical Observations." *Symbolic Interaction* 13, 2 (1990): 257–279.

Ehrenreich, Barbara. *The Hearts of Men: American Dreams and the Flight from Commitment.* Garden City, N.Y.: Anchor Press, 1983.

Ehrlich, Paul. *The End of Affluence.* New York: Ballantine, 1974.

Ehrman, John. *The Eighties: America in the Age of Reagan.* New Haven, Conn.: Yale University Press, 2005.

Englehardt, Tom. *The End of Victory Culture: Cold War America and the Disillusioning of a Generation.* New York: Basic Books, 1995.

Engs, Ruth Clifford. *Clean Living Movements: American Cycles of Health Reform.* Westport, Conn.: Praeger, 2000.

Ernst, Robert. *Weakness Is a Crime: The Life of Bernarr MacFadden.* Syracuse, N.Y.: Syracuse University Press, 1991.

Evans, Sara M. *Born for Liberty: A History of Women in America.* New York: Macmillan, 1989.

Ewing, Reid. "The Relationship between Urban Sprawl, Physical Activity, Obesity and Morbidity." *American Journal of Health Promotion* 18, 1 (September–October 2003): 47–57.

Fair, John D. *Muscletown USA: Bob Hoffman and the Manly Culture of York Barbell.* University Park: Pennsylvania University Press, 1999.

Featherstone, Mike, Mike Hepworth, and Bryan S. Turner, eds. *The Body: Social Process and Cultural Theory.* London: Sage Publications, 1991.

Filene, Peter G. Into the Arms of Others: A Cultural History of the Right-to-Die in America. Chicago: Ivan R. Dee, 1998.

Fineberg, Robert Gene. Jogging: The Dance of Death. Port Washington, N.Y.: Ashley Books, 1980.

Fixx, James F. The Complete Book of Running. New York: Random House, 1977.

Fleming, Thomas Michael. "The Aerobic Years: An Historical Analysis of the Work of Kenneth H. Cooper and His Influence Promoting Healthy Lifestyles." Ph.D. diss., Texas A&M, 1989.

Flint, Anthony. This Land: The Battle over Sprawl and the Future of America. Baltimore: Johns Hopkins University Press, 2006.

Foster, Mark S. A Nation on Wheels: The Automobile Culture in America since 1945. Belmont, Calif.: Thomson/Wadsworth, 2003.

Fox, Daniel M. Power and Illness. Berkeley: University of California Press, 1993.

Frank, Arthur W. "Bringing Bodies Back In: A Decade Review." Theory, Culture & Society 7 (1990): 131–162.

Friedan, Betty. The Feminine Mystique. New York: Norton, 1963.

Friedman, Meyer, and Ray H. Rosenman. Type A Behavior and Your Heart. New York: Knopf, 1974.

Friermood, Harold T. "Health Clubs in the YMCA with Respect to Current Status and Development of Operating Standards." Ed.D. diss., New York University, 1954.

Frum, David. How We Got Here: The 70s—The Decade that Brought You Modern Life (for Better or Worse). New York: Basic Books, 2000.

Fussell, Samuel. Muscle: Confessions of an Unlikely Bodybuilder. New York: Poseidon Press, 1991.

Gaines, Charles, and George Butler. Pumping Iron: The Art and Sport of Bodybuilding. New York: Simon & Schuster, 1974.

Geller, Alyson. "Smart Growth: A Prescription for Livable Cities." American Journal of Health Promotion 93, 9 (September 2003): 1410–1414.

Gelvin, E. Philip, and Thomas H. McGavack. Obesity: Its Cause, Classification and Care. New York: Hoeber-Harper, 1957.

Gertler, Menard. You Can Predict Your Heart Attack and Prevent It. New York: Random House, 1963.

Gilbert, James. A Cycle of Outrage: America's Reaction to the Juvenile Delinquent in the 1950s. New York: Oxford University Press, 1986.

Gillick, Muriel R. "Health Promotion, Jogging, and the Pursuit of the Moral Life." Journal of Health Politics, Policy and Law 9, 3 (Fall 1984): 369–387.

Gilman, Sander. Fat: A Cultural History of Obesity. Cambridge, U.K.: Polity Press, 2008.

———. *Fat Boys: A Slim Book.* Lincoln: University of Nebraska Press, 2004.

Glassner, Barry. *Bodies: Why We Look the Way We Do (and How We Feel about It).* New York: G. P. Putnam's Sons, 1988.

———. "Fitness and the Postmodern Self." *Journal of Health and Social Behavior* 30, 2 (June 1989): 180–191.

Gofman, John W. *What We Do Know about Heart Attacks.* New York: G. P. Putnam's Sons, 1958.

Goldstein, Michael S. *The Health Movement: Promoting Fitness in America.* New York: Twayne, 1992.

Gotaas, Thor. *Running: A Global History.* London: Reaktion Books, 2009.

Graebner, William. "America's *Poseidon Adventure.*" In *America in the 70s,* ed. Beth Bailey and David Farber, 157–180. Lawrence: University Press of Kansas, 2004.

———. *Coming of Age in Buffalo: Youth and Authority in the Postwar Era.* Philadelphia: Temple University Press, 1990.

———. "The 'Containment' of Juvenile Delinquency: Social Engineering and American Youth Culture in the Postwar Era." *American Studies* 27, 1 (1986): 81–98.

Graham, M. F. *Prescription for Life.* New York: David McKay, 1966.

Green, Harvey. *Fit for America: Health, Fitness, Sport and American Society.* Baltimore: Johns Hopkins University Press, 1988.

———. Introduction to *Fitness in American Culture: Images of Health, Sport and the Body, 1830–1940,* ed. Kathryn Grover, 3–17. Amherst: University of Massachusetts Press, 1989.

Griswold, Robert L. *Fatherhood in America: A History.* New York: Basic Books, 1993.

———. "The 'Flabby American,' the Body, and the Cold War." In *A Shared Experience: Men, Women and the History of Gender,* ed. Laura McCall and Donald Yacovone, 323–348. New York: New York University Press, 1998.

Grover, Kathryn, ed. *Fitness in American Culture: Images of Health, Sport and the Body, 1830–1940.* Amherst: University of Massachusetts Press, 1989.

Gustav-Wrathall, John Donald. *Take the Young Stranger by the Hand: Same-Sex Relations and the YMCA.* Chicago: University of Chicago Press, 1998.

Gutfreund, Owen. *Sprawl: Highways and the Reshaping of the American Landscape.* Oxford: Oxford University Press, 2004.

Guthman, Julie. *Weighing In: Obesity, Food Justice and the Limits of Capitalism.* Berkeley: University of California Press, 2011.

Hamlin, Richard E. *A New Look at YMCA Physical Education.* New York: Association Press, 1959.

Hansen, Kenneth K. *Heroes behind Barbed Wire.* Princeton, N.J.: Van Nostrand, 1957.

Hawley, Cameron. *The Hurricane Years.* Boston: Little, Brown, 1968.

Heady, J. A., J. N. Morris, and P. A. Raffle. "The Physique of London Busmen: The Epidemiology of Uniforms." *Lancet* 271, 6942 (September 15, 1956): 569–570.

Heissenberger, Klaus D. "An All-American Body? Bruce Springsteen's Working-Class Masculinity in the 1980s." In *The Embodiment of American Culture*, ed. Heinz Tschachler, Maureen Devine, and Michael Draxlbauer, 101–110. New Brunswick, N.J.: Transaction, 2003.

Henriksen, Margot A. *Dr. Strangelove's America: Society and Culture in the Atomic Age.* Berkeley: University of California, 1997.

Hertzberg, Hendrik. "The Short Happy Life of the American Yuppie." In *Culture in an Age of Money: The Legacy of the 1980s in America*, ed. Nicolaus Mills, 66–82. Chicago: Ivan R. Dee, 1990.

Heywood, Leslie. *Bodymakers: A Cultural Anatomy of Women's Body Building.* New Brunswick, N.J.: Rutgers University Press, 1998.

Hine, Thomas. *The Great Funk: Falling Apart and Coming Together (on a Shag Rug) in the Seventies.* New York: Sarah Crichton Books, 2007.

———. *Populuxe.* New York: Knopf, 1986.

Hoganson, Kristin. *Fighting for American Manhood: How Gender Politics Provoked the Spanish American and Philippine American Wars.* New Haven, Conn.: Yale University Press, 1998.

Hooven, F. Valentine. *Beefcake: The Muscle Magazines of America, 1950–1970.* Berlin: Taschen Verlag, 1996.

Hughes, Ellen Roney. "Machines for Better Bodies: A Cultural History of Exercise Machines, 1830–1950." Ph.D. diss., University of Maryland, 2001.

Hunt, William R. *Body Love: The Amazing Career of Bernarr MacFadden.* Bowling Green, Ohio: Bowling Green University Popular Press, 1989.

Hunter, Edward. *Brainwashing: The Story of Men Who Defied It.* New York: Farrar, Straus & Cudahy, 1956.

Hutchin, Kenneth C. *How Not to Kill Your Husband.* New York: Hawthorn Books, 1962.

Illich, Ivan. *Medical Nemesis: The Expropriation of Health.* New York: Pantheon, 1976.

Illick, Joseph E. *American Childhoods.* Philadelphia: University of Pennsylvania Press, 2002.

Ingham, Alan G. "From Public Issue to Personal Trouble: Well-Being and the Fiscal Crisis of the State." *Sociology of Sport Journal* 2 (1985): 43–55.

Jackson, Kenneth T. *Crabgrass Frontier: The Suburbanization of the United States.* Oxford: Oxford University Press, 1985.

Jamieson, Katherine M. "Reading Nancy Lopez." In *Reading Sport: Critical Essays on Power and Representation*, ed. Susan Birrell and Mary G. McDonald, 144–165. Boston: Northeastern University Press, 2000.

Jarvis, Christina S. *The Male Body at War: American Masculinity during World War II*. De Kalb: Northern Illinois University Press, 2004.

Jay, Kathryn. *More than Just a Game: Sports in American Life since 1945*. New York: Columbia University Press, 2004.

Jeffords, Susan. *Hard Bodies: Hollywood Masculinity in the Reagan Era*. New Brunswick, N.J.: Rutgers University Press, 1994.

Johnson, David K. "Physique Pioneers: The Politics of 1960s Gay Consumer Culture." *Journal of Social History* 43, 4 (Summer 2010): 867–892.

Johnson, Elmer. *The History of YMCA Physical Education*. Chicago: Association Press, 1979.

Johnson, Harry J. *Keeping Fit in Your Executive Job*. New York: American Management Association, 1962.

Johnson, Haynes. *Sleepwalking through History*. New York: Anchor Books, 1991.

Jolliffe, Norman, Seymour Rinzler, and Morton Archer. "The Anti-Coronary Club; Including a Discussion of the Effects of a Prudent Diet on the Serum Cholesterol Level of Middle-Aged Men." *American Journal of Clinical Nutrition* 7 (July–August 1959): 451–462.

Jou, Chin. "Controlling Consumption: The Origins of Modern American Ideas about Food, Eating, and Fat, 1886–1930." Ph.D. diss., Princeton University, 2009.

Kagan, Elizabeth, and Margaret Morse. "The Body Electronic: Aerobic Exercise on Video: Women's Search for Empowerment and Self-Transformation." *TDR, The Drama Review* 32, 4 (1988): 164–179.

Kasson, John. *Houdini, Tarzan and the Perfect Man: The White Male Body and the Challenge of Modernity in America*. New York: Hill & Wang, 2001.

Kaufman, David. *Shul with a Pool: The Synagogue Center in America*. Hanover, N.H.: University Press of New England, 1999.

Keats, John. *The Insolent Chariots*. Philadelphia: J. B. Lippincott, 1958.

———. *Schools without Scholars*. Boston: Houghton Mifflin, 1958.

Kimmel, Michael. *Manhood in America: A Cultural History*. New York: Free Press, 1996.

Kinkead, Eugene. *In Every War But One*. New York: Norton, 1959.

———. "A Reporter at Large: The Study of Something New in History." *New Yorker*, October 24, 1957, 114–169.

Knowles, John H. "Doing Better and Feeling Worse." *Daedalus* 106 (Winter 1977): 1–7.

Kolata, Gina. *Ultimate Fitness: The Quest for Truth about Health and Exercise*. New York: Farrar, Straus & Giroux, 2003.

Kuznick, Peter J., and James Gilbert, eds. *Rethinking Cold War Culture*. Washington, D.C.: Smithsonian Institution Press, 2001.

Lasby, Clarence G. *Eisenhower's Heart Attack: How Ike Beat Heart Disease and Held On to the Presidency*. Lawrence: University Press of Kansas, 1996.

Lasch, Christopher. *The Culture of Narcissism: American Life in an Age of Diminishing Expectations*. New York: Norton, 1978.

Lattin, Don. *Following Our Bliss: How the Spiritual Ideals of the Sixties Shape Our Lives Today*. San Francisco: HarperCollins, 2003.

Leavitt, Judith Walzer, and Ronald L. Number, eds. *Sickness and Health in America: Readings in the History of Medicine and Public Health*. Madison: University of Wisconsin Press, 1985.

Leichter, Howard M. *Free to Be Foolish: Politics and Health Promotion in the United States and Great Britain*. Princeton, N.J.: Princeton University Press, 1991.

Levenstein, Harvey. *Paradox of Plenty: A Social History of Eating in Modern America*. New York: Oxford University Press, 1993.

Levine, Martin P. *Gay Macho: The Life and Death of the Homosexual Clone*. New York: New York University Press, 1998.

Levy, Daniel, and Susan Brink. *A Change of Heart: How the Framingham Heart Study Helped Unravel the Mysteries of Cardiovascular Disease*. New York: Knopf, 2005.

Lewis, Michael. *The Money Culture*. New York: Norton, 1991.

Lloyd, Moya. "Feminism, Aerobics and the Politics of the Body." *Body and Society* 2, 2 (1996): 79–98.

Long, Ron. "The Fitness of the Gym." *Harvard Gay & Lesbian Review*, Summer 1997, 20–22.

Losano, Antonia, and Brenda A. Risch. "Resisting Venus: Negotiating Corpulence in Exercise Videos." In *Bodies out of Bounds: Fatness and Transgression*, ed. Jana Evans Braziel and Kathleen LeBesco, 111–129. Berkeley: University of California Press, 2001.

Love, Robert. *The Great Oom: The Improbable Birth of Yoga in America*. New York: Viking, 2010.

Lovegren, Sylvia. *Fashionable Food: Seven Decades of Food Fads*. New York: Macmillan, 1995.

Lowe, Maria R. *Women of Steel: Female Bodybuilders and the Struggle for Self-Definition*. New York: New York University Press, 1998.

Lowenberg, June S. *Caring and Responsibility: The Crossroads between Holistic Practice and Traditional Medicine*. Philadelphia: University of Pennsylvania Press, 1989.

Luciano, Lynne. *Looking Good: Male Body Image in America*. New York: Hill & Wang, 2001.

———. "Muscularity and Masculinity in the United States: A Historical Overview." In *The Muscular Ideal: Psychological, Social and Medical Perspectives*, ed. J. Kevin Thompson and Guy Cafri, 41–65. Washington, D.C.: American Psychological Association, 2007.

Lupton, Deborah. *The Imperative of Health*. London: Sage, 1995.

Lutz, Catherine. "Epistemology of the Bunker: The Brainwashed and Other New Subjects of Permanent War." In *Inventing the Psychological: Toward a Cultural History of Emotional Life in America*, ed. Joel Pfister and Nancy Schnog, 245–267. New Haven, Conn.: Yale University Press, 1997.

Lykins, Daniel L. *From Total War to Total Diplomacy: The Advertising Council and the Construction of the Cold War Consensus*. Westport, Conn.: Praeger, 2003.

Maguire, Jennifer Smith. *Fit for Consumption: Sociology and the Business of Fitness*. London: Routledge, 2008.

Maguire, Joseph, and Louise Mansfield. "'No-Body's Perfect': Women, Aerobics and the Body Beautiful." *Sociology of Sport Journal* 15 (1998): 109–137.

Mandell, Richard D. *Sport: A Cultural History*. New York: Columbia University Press, 1984.

Marling, Karal Ann. *As Seen on TV: The Visual Culture of Everyday Life in the 1950s*. Cambridge, Mass.: Harvard University Press, 1996.

Martin, Luther H., Huck Gutman, and Patrick H. Hutton, eds. *Technologies of the Self: A Seminar with Michel Foucault*. Amherst: University of Massachusetts Press, 1988.

Martin, Randy, and Toby Miller, eds. *Sportcult*. Minneapolis: University of Minnesota Press, 1999.

Marty, Myron A. "Pop Culture in the '80s: Plenty of Distractions." In *The 1980s*, ed. James D. Torr, 178–189. San Diego: Greenhaven Press, 2000.

May, Elaine Tyler. *Homeward Bound: American Families in the Cold War Era*. New York: Basic Books, 1988.

May, Kirse Granat. *Golden State, Golden Youth: The California Image in Popular Culture, 1955–1966*. Chapel Hill: University of North Carolina Press, 2002.

May, Lary, ed. *Recasting America: Culture and Politics in the Age of Cold War*. Chicago: University of Chicago Press, 1989.

McClarnand, Elaine, and Steve Goodson, eds. *The Impact of the Cold War on American Popular Culture*. Carrollton: State University of West Georgia, 1999.

McElroy, Mary. *Resistance to Exercise: A Social Analysis of Inactivity*. Champaign, Ill.: Human Kinetics, 2002.

McEnaney, Laura. *Civil Defense Begins at Home: Militarization Meets Everyday Life in the Fifties*. Princeton, N.J.: Princeton University Press, 2000.

McGee, Micki. *Self-Help, Inc.: Makeover Culture in American Life.* Oxford: Oxford University Press, 2005.

McKenzie, Shelly. "Athletic Clubs." In *Sports in America from Colonial Times to the Twenty-First Century: An Encyclopedia,* ed. Steven A. Riess. Armonk, N.Y.: Sharpe Online Reference, 2011.

————. "Weak Hearts and Wedding Day Figures: Exercise and Health Promotion in the 1960s." In *Women, Wellness and the Media,* ed. Margaret C. Wiley, 199–229. Newcastle, U.K.: Cambridge Scholars Press, 2008.

Melosh, Barbara. *Engendering Culture: Manhood and Womanhood in New Deal Public Art and Theater.* Washington, D.C.: Smithsonian Institution Press, 1991.

Messner, Michael A., and Donald F. Sabo. *Sex, Violence and Power in Sports.* Freedom, Calif.: Crossing Press, 1994.

Metzl, Jonathan M. "Why 'Against Health'?" In *Against Health: How Health Became the New Morality,* ed. Jonathan M. Metzl and Anna Kirkland, 1–11. New York: New York University, 2010.

Milio, Nancy. "The Profitization of Health Promotion." *International Journal of Health Services* 18, 4 (1988): 573–585.

Miller, Lori K., and Lawrence W. Fielding. "The Battle between the For-Profit Health Club and the 'Commercial' YMCA." *Journal of Sport and Social Issues* 19, 1 (February 1995): 76–107.

Mills, Nicolaus, ed. *Culture in an Age of Money: The Legacy of the 1980s in America.* Chicago: Ivan R. Dee, 1990.

Montez de Oca, Jeffrey. "'As Our Muscles Get Softer, Our Missile Race Becomes Harder': Cultural Citizenship and the Muscle Gap." *Journal of Historical Sociology* 18, 3 (September 2005): 145–172.

Moore, Kenny. *Bowerman and the Men of Oregon: The Story of Oregon's Legendary Coach and Nike's Cofounder.* Emmaus, Pa.: Rodale, 2006.

Moore, Pamela V., and Geraldine C. Williamson. "Health Promotion: Evolution of a Concept." *Nursing Clinics of North America* 19, 2 (June 1984): 195–206.

Morris, David. *Illness and Culture in the Postmodern Age.* Berkeley: University of California Press, 1998.

Morris, J. N., J. A. Heady, P. A. B. Raffle, C. G. Roberts, and J. W. Parks. "Coronary Heart Disease and Physical Activity of Work." *Lancet* 2 (1953): 1052–1057, 1111–1120.

Mozes, Eugene B. *Living beyond Your Heart Attack.* Englewood Cliffs, N.J.: Prentice-Hall, 1959.

Mrozek, Donald J. "The Cult and Ritual of Toughness in Cold War America." In *Rituals and Ceremonies in Popular Culture,* ed. Ray B. Browne, 178–191. Bowling Green, Ohio: Bowling Green University Popular Press, 1980.

————. *Sport and American Mentality, 1880–1910*. Knoxville: University of Tennessee Press, 1983.

Nestle, Marion. *Food Politics: How the Food Industry Influences Nutrition and Health.* Berkeley: University of California Press, 2002.

Oakes, Guy. *The Imaginary War: Civil Defense and American Cold War Culture.* New York: Oxford University Press, 1994.

Oldenburg, Ray. *The Great Good Place.* New York: Paragon House, 1989.

Olszewski, Todd. "Cholesterol: A Scientific, Medical and Social History, 1908–1962." Ph.D. diss., Yale University, 2008.

Osgerby, Bill. *Playboys in Paradise: Masculinity, Youth and Leisure-Style in Modern America.* Oxford: Berg, 2001.

Padurano, Dominique. "Making American Men: Charles Atlas and the Business of Bodies, 1892–1945." Ph.D. diss., Rutgers University, 2007.

Palladino, Grace. *Teenagers: An American History.* New York: HarperCollins, 1996.

Park, Roberta. "A Decade of the Body: Researching and Writing about the History of Health, Fitness, Exercise and Sport, 1983–1993." *Journal of Sport History* 21, 1 (Spring 1994): 59–82.

————. "History of Research on Physical Activity and Health: Selected Topics, 1867 to the 1950s." *Quest* 47 (1995): 274–287.

————. *Measurement of Physical Fitness: A Historical Perspective.* Washington, D.C.: U.S. Department of Health and Human Services, Public Health Service, 1988.

Pasley, Virginia. *21 Stayed: The Story of the American GIs Who Chose Communist China—Who They Were and Why They Stayed.* New York: Farrar, Straus & Cudahy, 1955.

Pate, Russell R. "The Evolving Definition of Physical Fitness." *Quest* 40 (1988): 174–179.

Peiss, Kathy. *Hope in a Jar: The Making of America's Beauty Culture.* New York: Metropolitan Books, 1998.

Pendergast, Tom. *Creating the Modern Man: American Magazines and Consumer Culture, 1900–1950.* Columbia: University of Missouri Press, 2000.

Pillsbury, Richard. *No Foreign Food: The American Diet in Time and Place.* Boulder, Colo.: Westview Press, 1998.

Plymire, Darcy. "A Moral Exercise: Long Distance Running in the 1970s." Ph.D. diss., University of Iowa, 1996.

Plymire, Darcy C. "Positive Addiction: Running and Human Potential in the 1970s." *Journal of Sport History* 31, 3 (2004): 297–316.

————. "Running, Heart Disease, and the Ironic Death of Jim Fixx." *Research Quarterly for Exercise and Sport* 73, 1 (2002): 38–46.

Pronger, Brian. *Body Fascism: Salvation in the Technology of Physical Fitness*. Toronto: University of Toronto Press, 2002.

Putney, Clifford W. "From Character to Body Building: The YMCA and the Suburban Metropolis, 1950–1980." In *Men and Women Adrift: The YMCA and the YWCA in the City*, ed. Nina Mjagkij and Margaret Spratt, 231–249. New York: New York University Press, 1997.

———. "Going Upscale: The YMCA and Postwar America, 1950–1990." *Journal of Sport History* 20, 2 (Summer 1993): 151–166.

———. *Muscular Christianity: Manhood and Sports in Protestant America, 1880–1920*. Cambridge, Mass.: Harvard University Press, 2001.

Rader, Benjamin G. *American Sports: From the Age of Folk Games to the Age of Televised Sports*. Upper Saddle River, N.J.: Prentice-Hall, 1983.

———. "The Quest for Self-Sufficiency and the New Strenuosity: Reflections on the Strenuous Life of the 1970s and 1980s." *Journal of Sport History* 18, 2 (Summer 1991): 255–266.

Reverby, Susan, and David Rosner, eds. *Health Care in America: Essays in Social History*. Philadelphia: Temple University Press, 1979.

Richards, Marc. "The Cold War's 'Soft' Recruits." *Peace Review* 10, 3 (September 1998): 435–441.

Roberts, Randy, and James S. Olson. "Perfect Bodies, Eternal Youth: The Obsession of Modern America." *Lamar Journal of the Humanities* 25, 1 (1989): 39–55.

———. *Winning Is the Only Thing: Sports in America since 1945*. Baltimore: Johns Hopkins University Press, 1989.

Rothstein, William G. *Public Health and the Risk Factor: A History of an Uneven Medical Revolution*. Rochester, N.Y.: University of Rochester Press, 2003.

Rotskoff, Lori. *Love on the Rocks: Men, Women, and Alcohol in Post–World War II America*. Chapel Hill: University of North Carolina Press, 2002.

Sabo, Don, and Sue Curry Jansen. "Seen But Not Heard: Images of Black Men in Sports Media." In *Sex, Violence and Power in Sports*, ed. Michael A. Messner and Donald F. Sabo, 150–160. Freedom, Calif.: Crossing Press, 1994.

Sabol, Blair. *The Body of America*. New York: Arbor House, 1986.

Sack, Daniel. *Whitebread Protestants: Food and Religion in American Culture*. New York: St. Martin's Press, 2000.

Salazar, James B. *Bodies of Reform: The Rhetoric of Character in Gilded Age America*. New York: New York University Press, 2010.

Sampson, Anthony. *Company Man: The Rise and Fall of Corporate Life*. New York: Random House, 1995.

Sassatelli, Roberta. *Fitness Culture: Gyms and the Commercialisation of Discipline and Fun.* London: Palgrave Macmillan, 2010.

Schaller, Michael. *Reckoning with Reagan: America and Its President in the 1980s.* New York: Oxford University Press, 1992.

Schulman, Bruce J. *The Seventies: The Great Shift in American Culture, Society, and Politics.* New York: Free Press, 2001.

Schumacher, E. F. *Small Is Beautiful: Economics as if People Mattered.* 1973. Reprint, New York: Harper & Row, 1989.

Schur, Edwin. *The Awareness Trap: Self-Absorption Instead of Social Change.* New York: McGraw-Hill, 1976.

Schuster, David. *Neurasthenic Nation: America's Search for Health, Happiness and Comfort, 1869–1920.* New Brunswick, N.J.: Rutgers University Press, 2011.

Schwartz, Hillel. *Never Satisfied: A Cultural History of Diets, Fantasies and Fat.* New York: Free Press, 1986.

Schwartz, Susan E. B. *Into the Unknown: The Remarkable Life of Hans Kraus.* New York: iUniverse, 2005.

Secretary of Defense's Advisory Committee on Prisoners of War. *POW: The Fight Continues after the Battle.* Washington, D.C.: U.S. Government Printing Office, 1955.

Seed, David. *Brainwashing: The Fictions of Mind Control.* Kent, Ohio: Kent State University Press, 2004.

Seid, Roberta Pollack. *Never Too Thin: Why Women Are at War with Their Bodies.* New York: Prentice Hall Press, 1989.

Selye, Hans. *The Stress of Life.* New York: McGraw-Hill, 1956.

Sewall, Gilbert T., ed. *The Eighties: A Reader.* Reading, Mass.: Addison-Wesley, 1997.

Sharp, Joanne P. *Condensing the Cold War: Reader's Digest and American Identity.* Minneapolis: University of Minnesota Press, 2000.

Signorile, Michaelangelo. *Life Outside: The Signorile Report on Gay Men: Sex, Drugs, Muscles, and the Passages of Life.* New York: HarperCollins, 1997.

Silverman, Debora. *Selling Culture: Bloomingdale's, Diana Vreeland and the New Aristocracy of Taste in Reagan's America.* New York: Pantheon, 1986.

Skolnick, Arlene. *Embattled Paradise: The American Family in an Age of Uncertainty.* New York: Basic Books, 1991.

Smith, James, Charles Gourgott, and Patrick Devine. "The Great Good Gym." In *Celebrating the Third Place,* ed. Ray Oldenburg, 130–140. New York: Marlowe, 2001.

Solomon, Henry A. *The Exercise Myth.* San Diego: Harcourt, Brace, Jovanovich, 1984.

Sonneborn, Robert M. *If Your Husband Has Coronary Heart Disease*. New York: Carlton Press, 1968.

Spears, Betty, and Richard A. Swanson. *History of Sport and Physical Activity in the United States*. Dubuque, Iowa: Wm. C. Brown, 1978.

Spielvogel, Laura. *Working out in Japan: Shaping the Female Body in Tokyo Fitness Clubs*. Durham, N.C.: Duke University Press, 2003.

Spigel, Lynn. *Make Room for TV: Television and the Family Ideal in Postwar America*. Chicago: University of Chicago Press, 1992.

Stanley, Gregory Kent. *The Rise and Fall of the Sportswoman: Women's Health, Fitness, and Athletics, 1860–1940*. New York: Peter Lang, 1996.

Starr, Paul. *The Social Transformation of American Medicine*. New York: Basic Books, 1982.

Stearns, Peter. *Fat History: Bodies and Beauty in the Modern West*. 2nd ed. New York: New York University Press, 2002.

Stein, Arthur. *Seeds of the Seventies: Values, Work, and Commitment in Post-Vietnam America*. Hanover, N.H.: University Press of New England, 1985.

Stein, Howard F. "Neo-Darwinism and Survival through Fitness in Reagan's America." *Journal of Psychohistory* 10, 2 (Fall 1982): 163–187.

Steinberg, Daniel. *The Cholesterol Wars: The Skeptics vs. the Preponderance of Evidence*. San Diego: Elsevier, 2007.

Stephens, Thomas. "Secular Trends in Adult Physical Activity: Exercise Boom or Bust?" *Research Quarterly for Exercise and Sport* 58, 2 (1987): 94–105.

Stern, Jane, and Michael Stern. *American Gourmet*. New York: HarperCollins, 1991.

Stern, Marc. "The Fitness Movement and the Fitness Center Industry, 1960–2000." Paper presented at the BHC annual meeting, 2008. Business and Economic History On-line.

———. "Real or Rogue Charity? Private Health Clubs vs. the YMCA, 1970–2000." Paper presented at the BHC annual meeting, 2011. Business and Economic History On-line.

Strasser, Susan. *Never Done: A History of American Housework*. 2nd ed. New York: Henry Holt, 2000.

Struna, Nancy. *People of Prowess: Sport, Leisure, and Labor in Early Anglo-America*. Urbana: University of Illinois, 1996.

Susman, Warren. *Culture as History: The Transformation of American Society in the Twentieth Century*. New York: Pantheon, 1984.

Swanson, B. S. "A History of the Rise of Aerobic Dance in the United States through 1980." M.A. thesis, San Jose State University, 1996.

Symon, Stefanie. *The Subtle Body: The Story of Yoga in America.* New York: Farrar, Straus & Giroux, 2010.

Tasker, Yvonne. *Spectacular Bodies: Gender, Genre and the Action Cinema.* London: Routledge, 1993.

Todd, Jan. "Bernarr MacFadden: Reformer of Feminine Form." *Journal of Sport History* 14, 1 (Spring 1987): 61–75.

Toon, Elizabeth, and Janet Golden. "'Live Clean, Think Clean, and Don't Go to Burlesque Shows': Charles Atlas as Health Advisor." *Journal of the History of Medicine* 57 (January 2002): 39–60.

Troy, Gil. *Morning in America: How Ronald Reagan Invented the 1980s.* Princeton, N.J.: Princeton University Press, 2005.

Turner, Bryan S. *The Body and Society.* 2nd ed. London: Sage Publications, 1996.

———. "Recent Developments in the Theory of the Body." In *The Body: Social Process and Cultural Theory,* ed. Mike Featherstone, Mike Hepworth, and Bryan S. Turner, 1–35. London: Sage Publications, 1991.

———. *Regulating Bodies: Essays in Medical Sociology.* London: Routledge, 1992.

U.S.D.A. Economics Research Service. "Major Trends in US Food Supply, 1909–1999." *Food Review* 23, 1 (January 2000): 1–15.

U.S. Department of Health, Education, and Welfare. *Healthy People: The Surgeon General's Report on Health Promotion and Disease Prevention.* Washington, D.C.: U.S. Government Printing Office, 1979.

U.S. Department of Health and Human Services. "Historical Background, Terminology, Evolution of Recommendations and Measurement." In *Physical Activity and Health: A Report of the Surgeon General,* 11–57. Washington, D.C.: U.S. Government Printing Office, 1996.

Verbrugge, Martha. *Able Bodied Womanhood: Personal Health and Social Change in 19th Century Boston.* New York: Oxford University Press, 1988.

Waldrep, Shelton, ed. *The Seventies: The Age of Glitter in Popular Culture.* New York: Routledge, 2000.

Walker, Susannah. *Style and Status: Selling Beauty to African American Women, 1920–1975.* Lexington: University Press of Kentucky, 2007.

Warner, John Harley, and Janet Tighe, eds. *Major Problems in the History of American Medicine and Public Health.* Boston: Houghton Mifflin, 2001.

Watson, Jonathan. *Male Bodies: Health, Culture and Identity.* Buckingham, U.K.: Open University Press, 2000.

Waxman, William W. "Physical Fitness Developments for Adults in the YMCA." In *Exercise and Fitness: A Collection of Papers Presented at the Colloquium on Exercise and Fitness,* 183–192. Monticello, Ill.: Athletic Institute, 1959.

Weisse, Allen B. *Heart to Heart: The Twentieth Century Battle against Cardiac Disease.* New Brunswick, N.J.: Rutgers University Press, 2002.

White, Philip G., and James Gillett. "Reading the Muscular Body: A Critical Decoding of Advertisements in *Flex* Magazine." *Sociology of Sport Journal* 11 (1994): 18–39.

White, Philip G., Kevin Young, and James Gillett. "Bodywork as a Moral Imperative: Some Critical Notes on Health and Fitness." *Loisir et Société* 18, 1 (1995): 159–182.

White, William L. *Captives of Korea: An Unofficial White Paper on the Treatment of War Prisoners: Our Treatment of Theirs, Their Treatment of Ours.* New York: Scribner, 1957.

Whitfield, Stephen J. *Culture of the Cold War.* 2nd ed. Baltimore: Johns Hopkins University Press, 1996.

Whorton, James. *Crusaders for Fitness: The History of American Health Reformers.* Princeton, N.J.: Princeton University Press, 1982.

———. *Nature Cures: The History of Alternative Medicine in America.* Oxford: Oxford University Press, 2002.

Whyte, William. *The Organization Man.* New York: Simon & Schuster, 1956.

Wiese, Andrew. *Places of Their Own: African American Suburbanization in the Twentieth Century.* Chicago: University of Chicago Press, 2004.

Wiggins, David K. "'Great Speed but Little Stamina': The Historical Debate over Black Athletic Superiority." In *The American Sport History,* ed. S. W. Pope, 312–338. Urbana: University of Illinois Press, 1997.

———. "The Notion of Double-Consciousness and the Involvement of Black Athletes in American Sport." In *Ethnicity and Sport in North American History and Culture,* ed. George Eisen and David K. Wiggins, 133–155. Westport, Conn.: Greenwood Press, 1994.

Wilkinson, Rupert. *American Tough: The Tough-Guy Tradition and American Character.* Westport, Conn.: Greenwood Press, 1984.

Willis, Susan. "Work(ing) Out." *Cultural Studies* 4, 1 (January 1990): 1–18.

Winkler, Mary G., and Letha B. Cole, eds. *The Good Body: Asceticism in Contemporary Culture.* New Haven, Conn.: Yale University Press, 1994.

Wolloch, Nancy. *Women and the American Experience.* New York: Knopf, 1984.

Wyden, Peter. *The Overweight Society.* New York: Pocket Books, 1965.

Zang, David W. *Sports Wars: Athletes in the Age of Aquarius.* Fayetteville: University of Arkansas Press, 2001.

Zingale, Donald P. "A History of the Involvement of the American Presidency in School and College Physical Education and Sports during the Twentieth Century." Ph.D. diss., University of Ohio, 1973.

———. "'Ike' Revisited on Sport and National Fitness." *Research Quarterly for Exercise and Sport* 48, 1 (1977): 12–18.

Zwieback, Adam J. "The 21 'Turncoat GIs': Nonrepatriations and the Political Culture of the Korean War." *Historian* 60 (Winter 1998): 345–362.

INDEX